MORTALITY AND OTHER
INVESTIGATIONS

VOLUME I

T0372340

MORTALITY AND OTHER INVESTIGATIONS

BY

H. W. HAYCOCKS, B.Sc.(Econ.), F.I.A.

AND

W. PERKS, F.I.A.

VOLUME I

CAMBRIDGE

Published for the Institute of Actuaries and the Faculty of Actuaries

AT THE UNIVERSITY PRESS

1955

CAMBRIDGE
UNIVERSITY PRESS

University Printing House, Cambridge CB2 8BS, United Kingdom

Cambridge University Press is part of the University of Cambridge.

It furthers the University's mission by disseminating knowledge in the pursuit of education, learning and research at the highest international levels of excellence.

www.cambridge.org
Information on this title: www.cambridge.org/9781316603635

© Cambridge University Press 1955

First published 1955
First paperback edition 2015

A catalogue record for this publication is available from the British Library

ISBN 978-1-316-60363-5 Paperback

CONTENTS

PREFACE

The subject of this book—Mortality and other Investigations—is divided between two sections of the examinations of the Institute of Actuaries. This division is in accordance with the principle of 'progressive approach' which was adopted for the new examination syllabus introduced after the Second World War and which has for its objective the parallel training of actuarial students in the three main classes of subjects making up the basic equipment of a qualified actuary: the mathematical subjects, pure and applied; the statistical subjects, general theory and actuarial applications; and the economic and financial subjects, including compound interest and investment of institutional funds. The first stage of the present subject for which this volume is intended to be the official reading is included in the second section of the statistical group of subjects along with the second stage of the general theory of statistics. The second stage of the present subject is included in the third section of the statistical subjects along with demography.

The scope and standard of the present volume are, therefore, determined by its purpose. With regard to scope the essential emphasis is on principles rather than a detailed treatment of investigations that have been made. The limits to its scope are defined negatively by reference to the examination syllabus—a detailed treatment of selection, of multiple decrements and of continuous exposed-to-risk formulae is not included. The standard of treatment is essentially determined by the normal equipment of the students for whose use the volume has been prepared. This includes elementary differential and integral calculus, algebraic probability, finite differences, elementary mathematical statistics and a first course in life and other contingencies. While every student using this book for his examinations will not necessarily by then have passed in all of these subjects the great majority will have read and sat for them in the examinations. A considerable equipment can, therefore, be assumed of the reader, although not all of it is required for present purposes.

Experience has shown over and over again that the real difficulty to the student in this subject is that for the most part his studies have hitherto all been in deductive subjects. For the first time he finds himself in the middle of a practical subject concerned with scientific observation and the mental processes of induction. Hitherto, for most of the problems that he has met there has been one answer to be logically deduced from the premises. Now there are vagueness, choice of procedure, approximation and decisions to be made that are directed to practical ends. Questions in test papers do not necessarily call for a specific answer—they often call for a discussion of pros and cons and the description of methods that are adequate, but not more than adequate, for the practical purposes to be served. The position of the student is the more difficult because he cannot fully weigh the significance of the practical purposes until a later date when his practical experience has reached a riper stage.

The exclusion of 'a detailed treatment of continuous exposed-to-risk formulae' has been very useful to us because it has forced us to abandon the traditional approach to the subject of exposed-to-risk by way of these formulae. The typical continuous exposed-to-risk formula is, after all, only a practical device that actuaries acquired in the embryonic stage of actuarial science. While in some circumstances it still plays a valuable part in practical work there is nothing fundamental about it, and a great deal of mortality and other investigation work goes on today without the use of continuous formulae. Then again, the traditional attitude to the census method is to treat it as something quite distinct from other methods. Our approach is to start from the simplest possible examples and to build up the subject from first principles by systematic stages embracing continuous and census formulae in the general development. For simplicity we have left the treatment of new entrants and withdrawals until the end, regarding these complications as little more than practical nuisances for which simple practical adjustments have to be made. The chapter on sickness and other rates follows the same general line except that for certain 'other rates', e.g. marriage and fertility rates, the reader is referred to P. R. Cox's *Demography* after a short general discussion of some of the special difficulties and statistical dangers in this field.

The first chapter contains a general discussion of the features of actuarial statistics. Some readers may find it preferable to leave this chapter until the end! Little need be said about the concluding chapters, two of which deal with simple graphical and finite-difference processes of graduation and construction of life tables. The last chapter describes the processes used in the construction of the more recent English Life Tables.

H.W.H.
W.P.

July 1955

CHAPTER I

INTRODUCTION

This book is about the principles and methods of actuarial statistics. By 'actuarial statistics' we mean the statistics that actuaries compile for the purposes of their professional work. Our subject is thus a severely practical one, and the methods used are such as are sufficient for the practical purposes to be served. Elaborate theoretical development would be inappropriate for our purpose; utilitarianism is the keynote and approximation pervades the whole subject. The modern developments of mathematical statistics have made hardly any impact in this field, partly because of this inevitable element of approximation, partly because small samples would be inappropriate for most of the practical purposes to be served and partly because the observed statistics in this field are subject to considerable variation, both from one group to another and at different times for the same group. Random variations affect the statistics of course, but the problems arising do not usually present themselves in the form of repeated samples from the same universe.

Actuarial statistics not only have to be compiled on sound principles to provide a solid bedrock of observational fact, but they have to be interpreted and adjusted and then often used only as a guide in fixing the statistical basis required for the solution of the practical problems in connexion with which they were compiled. These problems are nearly always concerned with the future, and to cope with them an actuary has to use his experienced judgment in setting up suitable hypotheses with regard to the future on the basis of his knowledge of observed statistical facts. It would, however, give a false indication of the actuary's work and function and of the claims that he makes for the value of his work to suggest that the hypotheses that he regards as suitable for his practical problems are often in any real sense intended to be close or even unbiased forecasts or estimates of the future. Occasionally a best shot—an educated guess—at future developments may be required, but for the most part the actuary's problems are arranged in such a way that the discrepancies between actual future fact and the prior assumptions regarding the future provide sources of profit or loss to the organization concerned or are absorbed in some system of periodical readjustment in the light of actual experience such as a bonus system in life assurance or an adjustment of the contribution rates in a pension fund following a valuation of assets and liabilities. It will be appreciated that the statistical aspects of an actuary's problems do not usually operate in isolation; these problems are nearly always financial and nearly always involve administration. Thus investment, interest rates and administrative expense come into the picture as well and, indeed, they not infrequently predominate in importance over the strictly statistical aspects.

A constant appreciation of this background to the actuary's statistical work is essential if this work and the methods used are to be kept in proper focus. We are concerned with the observational aspect of actuarial science—the appeal to statistical fact as the basis of sound procedure—but the approach is not on the lines of 'pure observation' that is found in certain sciences in which every little fact is grist to the mill. The observational processes of the actuary are nearly always directed to particular purposes, and they are organized in relation to conceptual models that have been developed from past experience and found useful as modes of procedure for analogous problems that have arisen before. The typical conceptual model used by the actuary is, of course, the mortality table which exhibits for a hypothetical population all of the same age x their subsequent life and death history, i.e. it shows how many out of l_x living at age x may be 'expected' to survive to the successive ages $x+1$, $x+2$, $x+3$ and so on, or what comes to the same thing, how many may be expected to die between ages x and $x+1$, between ages $x+1$ and $x+2$, and so on. The mortality table is thus a frequency (or probability) distribution of ages at death. Similarly, a 'service table' such as is used in connexion with certain types of pension schemes, expresses a frequency distribution of ages at withdrawal, at incapacity retirement and at normal retirement as well as ages at death in service.

When a surveyor makes certain measurements—lengths, angles and so on—he tacitly assumes a Euclidean model in which straight lines, circular arcs and other simple geometrical shapes are substituted for the obviously rough shapes that would more accurately describe the real situation. From the combination of his measurements and his Euclidean model the surveyor makes a number of logical deductions dependent upon his knowledge of mensuration based on Euclidean geometry and trigonometry, and he reaches certain propositions about his particular model which he then, without giving a moment's thought to the complicated logical structure of his procedure, treats as true propositions about the real situation. The rationale of this process depends for its justification and practical success on a trained ability to ignore those features of the real situation which are irrelevant to the final practical purpose of his work. The surveyor judges how far he can go in treating a curve or an irregular line as a straight line, or an angle of $87°$ as a right angle and so on; he makes approximations and reaches approximate answers. The validity of his work depends essentially upon his ultimate purpose.

When a rational gambler repeatedly gambles on the toss of a coin he adopts the conceptual model of a probability distribution represented by the binomial expression $(\frac{1}{2}+\frac{1}{2})^n$, and he is content to operate by analogy between the practical situation and the propositions logically deduced from the binomial model. He does not trouble to test the coin and tossing system for complete symmetry or to test the probability assumption that $p=\frac{1}{2}$ by a trial run of tosses subject to a significance test on the statistical result. He is content to assume the approximate basis that $p=\frac{1}{2}$ for his practical purpose and to abide by the consequences unless as a result of his experience he begins to suspect some kind of bias.

When a card player shuffles the pack of cards before dealing for a hand of bridge he is content with a limited shuffle. As a rational player he adopts as his conceptual model for determining his calls and play the assumption that the order of the cards in the pack is at random, and his experience tells him that this is a good enough approximation to the practical situation for his purpose.

In solo whist shuffling is forbidden. After each hand (with certain exceptions) the cards are gathered together, two cuts are made and then the cards are dealt in threes to the four players with a final singleton each, the last card dealt being turned up as trumps. The assumption of randomness in the order of the cards in the pack and in the deal would be a fatal assumption to make in these circumstances, and a player who made such an assumption would undoubtedly lose heavily against experienced players. The peculiar fascination of solo whist does in fact depend on the non-random distribution of the cards in the four hands. To play the game successfully a certain amount of experience is necessary to enable the player to gauge the effect on the distribution of the cards, of the absence of shuffling and of the form of dealing the cards. There is no conceptual model that can be appealed to for use in making bids and in playing the hand. No doubt statistics could be compiled of the biased distributions arising, but to carry out an adequate investigation would be an immense undertaking. In practice, players develop a very keen sense of the run of the cards, and are sometimes able to make a coup by assuming a distribution of certain cards highly relevant to success or failure which would be extremely unlikely on the random principles associated with ordinary whist or bridge as modified of course by the inferences to be drawn from the bids made and the play so far.

In the solution of financial problems involving future payments a conceptual model based on the assumption of a uniform rate of compound interest is often adopted leading to the typical exponential form for the value of a unit payable t years hence, viz. $e^{-t\delta}$. The actual interest earned each year may, or may not, in fact approximate to the amounts of interest assumed in the model.

A physicist knows that observation has established that a lump of radioactive material in constant conditions emits α-particles at a constant rate subject to random fluctuations. Apparently, the emission of particular particles cannot be foreseen, the observational facts being expressed by saying that the particles in a lump of radioactive material diminish in number according to the exponential probability distribution function Ne^{-at}, where a is the force of emission which is estimated by counting the number of particles emitted in a given period of time. The exponential function represents the conceptual model and a represents the parameter which when estimated from the observations enables the model to be fully described in numerical terms.

In many statistical problems a convenient and sufficiently accurate model to adopt is the normal distribution for which the two parameters—the mean and the standard deviation—have to be estimated in some suitable way.

The scientific approach of the actuary to his problems is very similar in principle to that used in all the other examples that have been given. In some respects it combines particular features from all of them, while in others it is considerably more complicated. There is usually a conceptual model—the idea of a mortality table or a service table—but the model is not usually defined in a specific form such as in surveying or in coin-tossing and bridge, nor does it often take an explicit mathematical form involving a few unknown parameters such as for radioactive material or in many ordinary statistical problems. Instead, each numerical term in the mortality or service table requires to be individually estimated, partly on the basis of observed statistics and partly by experienced judgment.

The subject of this book is the compilation and adjustment of the observed facts rather than the elucidation of the element of experienced judgment. If the conditions of human life remained unchanged over a long period, mortality tables for groups of people of various kinds could be compiled by the simple process of observing the life history of samples of these groups and then used either as they stand or after applying some kind of graduation process to remove, or to reduce, the random variations. Conditions of human life have not, however, remained unchanged, and there is no sign that they are likely to remain unchanged in the foreseeable future, and so a mortality table compiled in this way would be quite out of date by the time that it had been completed. Quite apart from this continual flux the simple process of counting the number dying at each subsequent age out of a number of lives chosen at a given age x would take a very long time to carry out—at least $100 - x$ years. Accordingly, instead of this process the early actuaries of the eighteenth and nineteenth centuries adopted the plan of observing groups of people of all ages over a short period of time and computing yearly mortality rates at each age from the observed numbers. After adjusting the observed rates to secure a smooth progression from age to age without altering their general level over short stretches of ages, they combined them together to form a mortality table by the process implied by the relations

$$p_x = 1 - q_x \quad \text{and} \quad l_{x+1} = p_x l_x,$$
$$l_{x+2} = p_{x+1} l_{x+1} = p_x p_{x+1} l_x,$$

and so on. Similar processes were adopted in building up service and other tables dependent on other contingencies of human life.

For some purposes and despite the doubt about the validity of the process, mortality and other tables are still built up in this way, while for other purposes attempts are made, on the basis of rates of mortality applicable to various earlier periods, to project rates that may be assumed to be appropriate for future periods and to build up models applicable to the future. A more simple purpose is often to compare the actual mortality of a group of lives in a given period with the number of deaths that would have occurred if the rates by some particular mortality table had in fact been closely experienced by the group during the period. Whatever may be the ultimate process to be used the essential starting point is to examine the mortality experience of one or more groups of lives. The typical measure of mortality is the ratio of the number of deaths occurring among a group of persons in a selected period of time; for example, E_x persons aged x are observed (exposed to risk) for a year, θ_x represents the number of such persons dying in the year and θ_x/E_x represents the rate of mortality.

This typical ratio illustrates the basic feature of all characteristic actuarial statistics. It may be expressed in general terms as the ratio of the number of times that a particular event occurs during a fixed period of time among a given group to the number of individuals in the group. This general expression of what we may call a time-rate is, in fact, too wide in its ambit for our purpose, because it includes many phenomena which would not normally come within the sphere of an actuary's work. It will be found, however, that the kind of examples that arise in other spheres rarely require more than a simple commonsense counting procedure which can be regarded as a special case of the more general processes used by actuaries. The more complicated processes of actuarial statistics have until fairly recent years usually been confined to the contingencies of human life, but the principles involved are of much wider application in theory, although the recognition of practical problems for this wider application has so far been relatively limited. However, the contingencies of human life, such as death, sickness, marriage, fertility, retirement and so on, which are the subject of actuarial treatment, nearly always exhibit a marked correlation in their incidence with age—and often with duration since the happening of some other contingency. Thus the incidence of death and of fertility both show considerable correlation with duration since marriage as well as with age. It is this correlation with age—and duration—that constitutes the special characteristic of the time-rates treated by actuaries. Age and duration themselves are both time characteristics, that is to say, they march forward together with the essential time element of the rates themselves. We might divide a group of lives into two subgroups according to, say, their sex, and then ascertain the mortality rates in a given year for the two sexes in the subgroups. If, on the other hand, we subdivided into ages and durations since entry into assurance a group of lives assured at a given point of time, we should not only have to fix successive ranges of ages and durations for the purpose of the subdivision but we should have to cope with the fact that as we observe the lives through the period of the investigation (e.g. a year) so would their ages and durations steadily progress. There is no doubt that as adult lives get older, so, on the average, does their health deteriorate and their mortality rates increase. Similarly, a group of lives, all of whom have passed a medical examination, steadily deteriorate, on the average, as the duration since the examination progresses. There is obviously a kind of progression towards destruction which is manifest throughout nature. The degree and rate of deterioration and the consequent level of mortality rates are affected by environmental features, and it is changes in these features and their effects that create the need for mortality investigations to be made at frequent intervals.

From a statistical point of view death is a simple event because it happens only once to an individual and must happen some time to every individual. It operates to remove the individual from the group of living persons—it is a 'decremental' phenomenon. Actuarial statistics are often concerned with events which operate as decrements, but they are by no means confined to decremental events. Some decremental events are reversible, e.g. a revival of a life policy is a negative lapse. Some events which are not decremental or reversible are repetitive. For example, in a sickness investigation the event is a day's sickness, and any individual may be the subject of one or more days of sickness in the period of the investigation. Fertility is even more complicated; multiple births take place—twins, triplets, etc.—but after a maternity a woman cannot normally again have a child until about 10 or 11 months have expired. This does not rigorously apply to a man—although it does sufficiently in practice—because he could have another child by another woman.

These various features of the events that are the subject of the various time-rates investigated by actuaries are important in interpreting the observed statistics and in adapting them for practical purposes. In particular, they require to be taken into account in considering the nature and level of the random element in the observed rates which we shall now briefly discuss. It is, of course, through the random element that the subject of actuarial statistics is connected with the general theory of mathematical statistics.

For mortality rates it is often useful to assume that the mortality rate for a given year of a group of persons aged x at the beginning of the year is a binomial variate generated by the binomial distribution $(p_x + q_x)^{E_x}$, where p_x and q_x are 'ideal' survival and mortality rates, so that the observed mortality rate is equal to q_x plus a random variable, of mean zero and variance $p_x q_x / E_x$. We need not assume that all the E_x lives are subject to identical probabilities of death like a set of symmetrical dice with $(q_x)^{-1}$ equally likely sides. All we need to do is to assume that E_x is a random sample from a hypothetical population (subject to a mortality rate of q_x) of sufficiently large numbers so that the extraction of E_x from the population makes no material difference to the mortality rate of the remainder. This avoidance of the assumption of homogeneity is not only more realistic than the dice model but leaves room for the development of an adequate theory of selection such as is required in life assurance and annuity mortality statistics, and in a reversed form in the mortality statistics of persons who have retired on incapacity pension. The validity of the assumption of binomiality of mortality rates, in the absence of certain disturbing features that are referred to later, is supported by the success attendant upon many examples of graduation of mortality rates.

The object of the process of graduation is to smooth the progression of the rates from age to age. That is the practical aim. The theoretical basis is the assumption that each rate contains a random error and that, shorn of these errors, the rates would show a smooth progression from age to age. Smoothness is a concept that has eluded a precise and generally accepted mathematical definition, but for actuarial purposes it usually means that the successive differences of the function concerned diminish and that third differences are small. Assuming that a particular graduation has succeeded in achieving smoothness the results can be tested for ' departure from the observed rates' (such a test may also be referred to as a 'test of fidelity' to the observed rates, although it would be more logical to refer to the closeness of the observed rates to the graduated rates which are, for the purpose of the test, being assumed to be 'true'). The process is to assume that the random errors in the observed rates are binomial and independent of each other. It is possible to devise various significance tests such that if the graduation survives the test, not only is the graduation judged acceptable but the assumption of binomiality is also supported.

The kind of disturbing features referred to above are the duplication of lives in an experience when an investigation of death claims under life policies is made without excluding the second, third, fourth, etc., policies on the same life. The existence of duplicates increases the variance of the random errors, and a correction of the significance test for this disturbance is always necessary when duplicates have not been eliminated. Various writers have discussed the subject. Redington and Michaelson (*Trans. 12th Int. Congr. Actu.*) provided a measure of the extent of the departure of the variances from the binomial variances including the effect of duplicates, and R. H. Daw (*J.I.A.* **72**, 174) has discussed the application of the measure in detail. Perks (*J.I.A.* **75**, 31) has suggested that a measure of the effect of duplicates alone could be obtained by taking a random sample of the deaths and ascertaining from them the proportion of lives in the investigation at each age with 1, 2, 3, etc., policies each. From these figures an estimate of the effect on the variances could easily be made (see, for example, *J.I.A.* **75**, 75, Beard and Perks).

A minor feature which affects the validity of the binomial assumption is the treatment of new entrants and withdrawals in computing the exposed-to-risk and ascertaining the deaths. If E_x is the computed exposed-to-risk, the number of lives contributing to E_x may be considerably greater than E_x because fractions of a year's exposure will have been accorded to the new entrants and withdrawals in the year. In the limit, if the number of lives contributing to E_x was very great, the average period of exposure in the year for each life being very small, the sampling distribution would tend to the Poisson limit. For example, if E_x were made up of nE_x lives all exposed for $1/n$ of a year each and subject to a rate of mortality of q_x/n, the binomial variance of the number of deaths $(nE_x)(q_x/n)(1 - q_x/n)$ would be insignificantly different from the Poisson variance $E_x q_x$. Since $E_x p_x q_x \doteq E_x q_x$ when q_x is not very large, the prevalence of fractional exposures suggests that the Poisson variance (subject to adjustment for duplicates) might as well always be used in mortality investigations. Care needs to be exercised, however, at the extreme old ages where p_x becomes significantly smaller than unity so that the binomial and Poisson variances depart significantly from each other.

In other cases when the event is not a simple once-for-all event like death, the sampling variance will be correspondingly modified. An example of this is given in Chapter 6 in connexion with sickness rates where the variance is obtained from the frequency distribution of durations of sickness. In the case of sickness, however, the assumption of independence between the rates at successive ages is probably seriously inappropriate. This applies with particular force to the 'all-periods' sickness and with less force to the rates for the separate periods.

We have already mentioned the possibility of sampling the deaths to estimate the distribution of duplicates. A mortality investigation based on a sample of the lives in the group under consideration would usually mean a too drastic reduction in the number of deaths observed. Mortality rates are small, and a large number of lives is required if rates at successive ages, free from too large random errors, are to be obtained. A thousand deaths spread over 50 ages means 20 deaths per age on the average, and a random error of about 20% of the mortality rate at each age on the average. If, for example, the average mortality rate is 1%, a thousand deaths requires a total exposed-to-risk of 100,000. It will be seen, therefore, that there is not much scope for useful random sampling in the ordinary sense. The suggestion has, however, been made that little would be lost in the precision of the mortality rates by taking a random sample of the exposed-to-risk in order to distribute the total exposed (either the actual known total or an estimated total based on the sampling fraction) approximately over the individual ages provided that all the deaths were recorded at their proper ages. This procedure would be otiose if the exposed-to-risk figures in ages were obtainable from statistics for the whole group compiled for some other purpose, e.g. for an actuarial valuation of liabilities.

CHAPTER 2

ONE-YEAR GROUP MORTALITY RATES

2·1. The choice of time-interval

Suppose that for some purpose it is desired to ascertain the rate of mortality experienced by a particular group of lives. This statement of objective is necessarily vague at this stage, but it will acquire greater precision as the discussion proceeds. The first thing to decide is the time-interval for the rate, that is, the period of time to which the rate of mortality relates. Time is of the essence of the matter because, in general, the longer the period of time the greater the rate will be. It is obvious that any period of time could be selected as the time-interval, but there are practical reasons for choosing a year and this is the general practice, except in certain special circumstances which we need not go into here.

One overwhelming reason for choosing a year as the time-interval—in addition to the influence of such conventions as yearly birthdays, yearly accounting and so on—is that, in temperate climes, mortality varies with the seasons, heavier in winter and lighter in summer, so that a year's mortality provides an average of the seasonal variation. In actual fact, some winters are exceptionally severe and some, whether severe or not, are marked by influenza epidemics; fortunately, in Great Britain other types of seasonal epidemics, such as the summer epidemics of poliomyelitis, do not, at the present time, cause sufficient deaths to make any significant impact on the general death-rate. Although a single calendar year may not be representative enough to provide a sufficient degree of averaging of the seasonal variation in mortality, this consideration will be ignored for the time being, and so also will the phenomenon of the trend in mortality over a period of years. For the present it will be assumed that mortality does not vary with time or fluctuate with the seasons.

2·2. A calendar-year experience

Having decided to investigate the rate of mortality for a year of a particular group of lives, the next thing to do is to select the particular year for the investigation. We could choose a particular calendar year from 1 January to 31 December inclusive, or we could start on any other date of the year from, say, 15 March of one year to 14 March of the next year. In either case the obvious thing to do would be to count the number of lives in the group on the starting date (e.g. 1 January) and then count the number of deaths occurring among the group during the ensuing year. It is assumed, for the present, that no fresh lives enter the group during the year and that none leave otherwise than by death. The ratio of the number of deaths to the number starting the year thus provides a crude death-rate analogous to the rate of mortality q in a mortality table, except that we are not yet distinguishing the lives by age.

Another form of mortality rate could be obtained by taking the ratio of the number of deaths to the average number living during the year. On the assumption that the deaths are reasonably uniformly spread over the year, an approximation to this 'mean population' (or to the 'population' in the middle of the year) can be obtained by deducting one-half of the number of deaths from the number starting the year. The resulting rate is what is known as a 'central rate' and is in a form analogous to the central mortality rate m in a mortality table, except that again we are not distinguishing the lives by age.

For the central rate we could equally well count the population in the middle of the year, or at the end of the year and add one-half of the deaths, or take the average of the number at the beginning, in the middle and at the end of the year. It will be appreciated that if we knew the number living at the beginning of the year and also the number of deaths during the year, we could compute the number living at the end of the year, and vice versa. But this would not apply if there were new entrants or leavers during the year.

2·3. A life-year experience

We now consider an alternative form of year for tracing the lives and ascertaining the deaths. This is the year from the birthday of each individual in a given calendar year to the birthday in the following year. Thus, although the time-interval is still a year, the investigation stretches over two calendar years, each individual being observed over only a single year of life. This process is, of course, a little artificial when we are not distinguishing the lives by age, but it would be a most natural procedure if we were so distinguishing them.

For the denominator of the mortality rate in the form analogous to q of the mortality table, we obviously require to know the number of lives reaching their respective birthdays in the first of the two calendar years over which the investigation extends. Then on the assumption, similar to that made when we were considering an experience over a calendar year, that *between birthdays* there are no new entrants to the group or leavers other than the deaths, the q-type of mortality rate is simply the ratio of the number of deaths between the respective birthdays to the total of those reaching their birthdays in the first of the two calendar years.

To obtain the central rate analogous to m of the mortality table, there are various possibilities. We could deduct one-half of the number of deaths from the total of those reaching their birthdays in the first calendar year to obtain the central exposed-to-risk, i.e. the denominator of the central rate; or we could count the lives reaching their birthdays in the second of the two calendar years and add one-half of the number of deaths; or we could count the lives in the group on 1 January of the second of the two calendar years and regard this as the mean population in the group *between* the two birthdays; or we could average this census total with the numbers in the group on their respective birthdays in each of the two years and treat the result as the mean population.

It is worth noting that this last process could be applied in two different ways. We could either take as the mean population one-third of the three totals (i.e. the number reaching their birthdays in the first calendar year, the number reaching 1 January of the second calendar year and the number reaching their birthdays in the second calendar year) or we could take as the mean population the mean between (a) the mean of the two birthday censuses and (b) the census on the intervening 1 January. There is no reason to suppose that (*a*) and (*b*) would be identical, although the suitability of the whole process of averaging or deducting one-half of the number of deaths from the first birthday census to obtain the central exposed-to-risk presupposes that the number of deaths from the first birthday to the end of the first calendar year is approximately the same as the number in the second calendar year before the second birthday, or, more generally, that the deaths are sufficiently uniformly spread over the period. There is a relevant complication arising out of the seasonal variation of mortality, but this need not detain us at this stage. If the mortality rate for the group is small, e.g. less than 2 or 3 %, the error in the mean population, and hence in the central mortality rate, which results from assuming a uniform distribution of deaths when they are not uniformly distributed, is not likely to be very serious.

2·4. A policy-year experience

We now come to a third form of year for tracing the lives and ascertaining the deaths. This form is especially important in connexion with some forms of investigation into the mortality of assured lives or annuitants in a life office. It could be used for any group where the anniversaries of the date of joining some organization or of reaching some relevant status, such as marriage or promotion to a higher grade of employment, are significant events in relation to the purposes for which the mortality investigation is being undertaken. For assured lives, the year in question is usually from the policy anniversary in one calendar year to the policy anniversary in the next calendar year, and the deaths required are those occurring between these two policy anniversaries. Here again, while the time-interval is one year the period of the investigation extends over two calendar years.

At the present stage of the discussion in which the lives are being considered as a whole in one single group, without distinction of age or duration since entry into insurance, the process of using policy anniversaries is identical with that of using birthdays, and the previous discussion on a life-year investigation applies identically with the substitution throughout of the words 'policy anniversary' for 'birthday'. When we come in the next chapter to introduce subdivisions of the population and deaths according to age and duration the divergence of the two processes will become apparent.

2·5. Subdivision of the group

Experience has shown that all kinds of factors affect mortality. Significant differences in the rate of mortality are found when a group of lives is divided into subgroups according to various characteristics, and this applies even when the rates are analysed also by age. In such circumstances a desirable course would be to try to isolate the effect of each characteristic by comparing subgroups in which all the other features are similar. This is in fact not possible partly because the subgroups become too small and partly because there are widespread correlations between the various relevant characteristics. For example, if the sexes are separated it is found that the two groups are differently distributed among the various occupations. Similarly, when a group of lives is subdivided into different occupation groups it is found that there are significant differences in the geographical distributions within the subgroups and in the distributions between town and country.

Apart from separating the sexes, this kind of division of the lives is not often a very relevant proceeding for actuarial purposes, but it is commonly made in the census publications for the population as a whole, and it undoubtedly has important significance from a sociological point of view. Such characteristics as sex, marital status, occupation, geographical area of residence, social class and so on, may be regarded as permanent or semi-permanent features, and, accordingly, subdivision by one or more of such characteristics does not raise any questions of principle; each subgroup may be regarded as a separate group on its own. Any individual passing from one group to another during the period of the investigation may be treated as a leaver from the old group and as a new entrant to the new group; the appropriate adjustments for new entrants and leavers generally are discussed in Chapter 5.

It will be seen later that the use of a method of mean populations automatically makes allowance for new entrants and leavers and, accordingly, there is a danger of their being overlooked, but in interpreting the results the realization that such movements take place and have in fact occurred in the population before the period of the investigation commences is often of considerable importance. For example, the mortality experience (even when analysed by age) of a group of men working as coal-miners in Kent would be an unsuitable basis for assessing premium rates for a group of men who at the time of entry happened to be coal-miners in Kent. Such an experience might, however, be relevant to a friendly society or pension fund, membership of which was confined to coal-miners in Kent, if the rules provided that men leaving the industry must leave the society or fund, although in such a case a mortality investigation confined to the members of the society or fund would be a more suitable basis for actuarial purposes.

2·6. Age and duration

Perhaps the most important factors affecting mortality are age and duration since 'selection'. By 'selection' is here meant the process of passing lives for inclusion in a group after some test of health. Such a test might be an actual medical examination for a life assurance policy or for entry into some particular occupation, or the passing of a questionnaire test as in non-medical life assurance; or it might be a self-imposed test, such as occurs when a man decides to purchase an annuity on his own life; or it might work in the reverse direction by picking out impaired lives, such as occurs in pension-fund work when a life enters the pensioners' group by reason of permanent disability. It should be noted here that the word 'selection' is often used in a very technical sense as meaning the *effect* on the mortality rates of a selecting process such as we have just described.

Age and duration are two characteristics of a very special kind in mortality investigation work, quite apart from the obvious fact that mortality rates vary greatly with age (from one or two per thousand per annum in some experiences at the young adult ages to over 50 % per annum in extreme old age), and also with duration (in some experiences being as low for the first year of duration as 40 % of the corresponding rate for the longer durations for the same attained age). The special point to which attention is being drawn is that both age and duration are measured in time units. They vary continuously throughout the period of the investigation, and it is this fact that creates the necessity for special treatment in mortality investigations. Indeed, it is largely the variety of ways in which these 'time' variables may be treated that is the subject of the first part of this book. A more detailed treatment of the same features will form the subject of the first part of the second volume of *Mortality and Other Investigations*.

Mortality experiences are often summarized in groups of ages and groups of durations. Rates may be shown and appropriately defined for quinary or denary age-groups and for the first few years of duration separately and for all durations thereafter together. In fact, the investigation itself may be made for such subgroups without further subdivision into individual ages or individual durations after, say, 3 or 5 years.

2·7. Summary

The first part of this chapter has been confined to a preliminary discussion of the simple problem of investigating the mortality of a group of lives as a single group over a single year, and some important principles have been illustrated. This was followed by a discussion of some general considerations bearing on the subdivision of the data leading to the conclusion that age and duration require special treatment. The next chapter will be concerned with subdivision of the data by age and duration. It will still be assumed that the investigation is confined to the deaths occurring in a single year among the lives in the group at the beginning of the year. The following chapter will extend the discussion to investigations over a series of years, still on the assumption that the mortality is not steadily rising or falling over the period. This discussion will include the principles of continuous exposed-to-risk formulae but without a detailed treatment. This will be followed in the succeeding chapter by an examination of the problems created by new entrants and leavers during the period of the investigation, and the usual approximate solutions will be indicated and embodied in the general process of the continuous formulae.

CHAPTER 3

ONE-YEAR MORTALITY RATES ANALYSED BY AGE AND BY DURATION

3·1. Subdivision by age—life-year investigation

In the last chapter we considered various ways of ascertaining the mortality rate of a group of lives over a period of 1 year without distinguishing the lives in any way. We now proceed to extend the problem by distinguishing the lives according to age so that mortality rates according to age may be obtained. In principle, the problem remains unaltered because we can subdivide the lives according to some definition of integral age, such as nearest integral age or age last birthday, and then regard each subgroup as a separate group for which the mortality rate—q or m—is required. For a life-year investigation this is, indeed, the position not only in principle but in practical application, because all we need to do for each age x is to count the lives reaching their xth birthdays in the first calendar year and record the corresponding deaths at each age x last birthday between the two birthdays. However, even for a life-year investigation we have a problem to decide if the exposed-to-risk figures are to be based on a census on 1 January of the second calendar year. On this date the ages of the lives will not, in general, be integral.

An obvious course would be to record the number in the population on 1 January at each age last birthday. Then, by adding to the number aged x last birthday at that date one-half of the number dying at age x last birthday between the two birthdays, we could obtain an approximation to the number of living at age x on their birthdays in the first calendar year. Alternatively, the exact number living on their birthdays could be obtained by dividing the number of deaths at age x last birthday into two groups, those dying in the first calendar year after their birthdays and those dying in the second calendar year before their birthdays. Then by adding the number in the first group of deaths to the number living at age x last birthday on 1 January we could obtain the exact number attaining age x in the first calendar year to form the denominator for the q-type of rate.

For the central rate we could approximate to the mean population by counting the number reaching age x on their birthdays in the first calendar year and deducting half of the total number of deaths at age x last birthday between the two birthdays. Alternatively, by deducting such of those deaths as occurred in the first calendar year we should reach the census figure at 1 January at age x last birthday which could be used as the mean population to form the denominator of the central rate.

3·2. Notation

It will be helpful to express the various processes in mathematical symbols, and we accordingly introduce here an *ad hoc* notation. For the purpose of exposition expressions in the form of the integral calculus will be used as a kind of shorthand to represent summations, but in so doing it is not intended to imply, unless expressly stated, that any of the functions are differentiable or even continuous. In response to any objection that this is a misuse of recognized mathematical symbolism it may be mentioned that strict orthodoxy can be secured by interpreting all the integrals in this book as Stieltjes integrals.

We now define $_tP_x$ as the number in the group at age x last birthday at time t, measuring t in years from the beginning of the first calendar year. We also write $_t\overset{o}{l}_{x+r}dr$ for the number aged $x+r$ to $x+r+dr$ at time t, the small 'o' above this and other symbols being used, as in *Statistics* by Johnson and Tetley, to mean that the numbers represented by the symbol are observed numbers and not the analogous functions of a mortality table; it will also serve as a warning that the various relations which connect the various symbols of a mortality table do not necessarily apply to the observed numbers.

We then have
$$\int_0^1 {}_1\overset{o}{l}_{x+r}dr = {}_1P_x,$$

representing the number living at age x last birthday on 1 January of the second calendar year.

Since r and t are measured in the same time-units we may also sum $_tl_x$ with respect to t from 0 to 1 and so obtain the number reaching age x in the first calendar year, viz.

$$\int_0^1 {}_tl_x\,dt = l_{(x)}.$$

The symbol $l_{(x)}$ is given no prefix because it does not refer to the living at a point of time; instead, the brackets round x are intended to indicate that x is the age at entry into the experience. Consistently with this we write

$$\int_1^2 {}_tl_{x+1}\,dt = l_{(x)+1}$$

for the number attaining age $x+1$ in the second calendar year. $l_{(x)+1}$ is, of course, to be distinguished from $l_{(x+1)}$ which is the number reaching age $x+1$ in the first calendar year.

Although at a later stage a more extensive notation for the deaths will be introduced it is sufficient for the present to symbolize the deaths at age x last birthday between the two birthdays by θ_x.

The symbols θ_x^α and θ_x^β are respectively used for the deaths after their birthdays in the first calendar year and for the deaths before their birthdays in the second calendar year, so that

$$\theta_x^\alpha + \theta_x^\beta = \theta_x.$$

It will be observed that

$$l_{(x)+1} = l_{(x)} - \theta_x,$$

which has an obvious analogy with the corresponding relation for the mortality table, because $l_{(x)+1}$ represents the actual survivors out of $l_{(x)}$, and accordingly we write $l_{(x)+s} = \int_s^{1+s} {}_tl_{x+s}\,dt$ for the number surviving to age $x+s$ out of $l_{(x)}$. But such analogies are rarely applicable to the observational symbols because these usually refer to cross-sections of many generations of different sizes rather than to the life history of a single generation. For example, $l_{(x+1)} \neq l_{(x)} - \theta_x$. Moreover, when new entrants and leavers are included in the scheme of things even the above analogous relationship ceases to apply.

3·3. Application of symbolism to a life-year investigation

We may now write down some relevant identities and approximations for a life-year investigation for 1-year rates based on the exposure and deaths between two birthdays:

$$\mathring{q}_x = \theta_x / \mathring{l}_{\{x\}}$$
$$= \theta_x / (\mathring{l}_{\{x\}+1} + \theta_x)$$
$$= \theta_x / ({}_1P_x + \theta_x^\alpha)$$
$$\doteqdot \theta_x / ({}_1P_x + \tfrac{1}{2}\theta_x),$$

$$\mathring{m}_x = \theta_x \Big/ \int_0^1 \mathring{l}_{\{x\}+s}\, ds$$
$$\doteqdot \theta_x / {}_1P_x$$
$$\doteqdot \theta_x / (\mathring{l}_{\{x\}} - \theta_x^\alpha)$$
$$\doteqdot \theta_x / (\mathring{l}_{\{x\}} - \tfrac{1}{2}\theta_x).$$

Since at all except the very advanced ages θ is small in relation to l, the difference between using θ^α and $\tfrac{1}{2}\theta$ in the denominators of $\mathring{q}$ and $\mathring{m}$ is of very little significance. Errors in the deaths in the numerators, on the other hand, have a direct effect on the results.

3·4. A calendar-year investigation

For a calendar-year investigation we are forced to use approximations both for the q-type and for the m-type of rates because the ages of the lives at the beginning, middle and end of the calendar year of the experience are not, in general, integral. The first thing to do is to decide on the method of distributing the lives over the ages, remembering that the usual objective is to obtain a set of mortality rates which may be taken as applying to the succession of integral ages. An obvious procedure would be to group the lives according to nearest integral age x, that is to say, all the lives whose exact age on 1 January was between $x - \tfrac{1}{2}$ and $x + \tfrac{1}{2}$ would be considered as a subgroup, and the deaths during the ensuing calendar year out of this subgroup would be counted. The resulting ratio would be the q-type of rate applicable to this particular subgroup of the lives. If the distribution of the lives on 1 January over the age-range $x - \tfrac{1}{2}$ to $x + \tfrac{1}{2}$ was approximately uniform, which would be the usual position since birthdays are commonly spread throughout the calendar year, the average age of the group on 1 January would be approximately x, and we could take the q for the subgroup as being an approximation to the rate of mortality for the integral age x. For the corresponding rates of the m-type we could deduct one-half of the number of deaths recorded at age x from the living recorded at age x to form the appropriate denominators. Alternatively, a census on 1 July according to ages last birthday would automatically provide the relevant denominators, because age x last birthday on 1 July is identical with nearest age x on the preceding 1 January.

An alternative grouping on 1 January would be according to age $x - 1$ last birthday, that is to say, all the lives whose exact age on 1 January was between $x - 1$ and x would be considered as a subgroup, and the deaths among these lives during the calendar year would be counted. This method of grouping would be suitable if the only information about age was the calendar year of birth. The resulting ratio would be the q-type of rate for this subgroup of the lives, but assuming that the lives on 1 January were more or less uniformly distributed over the age-range $x - 1$ to x, we could take the q for the subgroup as being an approximation to $\mathring{q}_{x-\frac{1}{2}}$.

Similarly, the ratio of the number of deaths to the mean number living over the calendar year would provide an approximation to $\mathring{m}_{x-\frac{1}{2}}$. The mean number living over the year could be obtained approximately by deducting half the number of deaths from the number living at age $x - 1$ last birthday on 1 January or by taking a census on 1 July of all those reaching their xth birthdays in the current calendar year, or by taking the mean between the number living at age $x - 1$ last birthday on 1 January and the number living at age x last birthday on 1 January of the following year.

In the earlier literature the difference between the calendar year of death and the calendar year of birth is referred to as the 'mean age' at death. This is an unfortunate piece of nomenclature, but a label is required and we shall accordingly use the phrase 'calendar-year age' for the difference between the current calendar year (of death, entry, withdrawal, etc.) and the calendar year of birth. If the calendar-year age at death is x, then the age on 1 January of the year of death is $x-1$ last birthday; hence the ratio of the number of deaths at calendar-year age x to the population on 1 January at age $x-1$ last birthday provides an approximation to $\mathring{q}_{x-\frac{1}{2}}$.

The deaths at calendar-year age x include lives whose exact ages at death range from $x-1$ to $x+1$, since a person born in January may die in December while a person born in December may die in January. Similarly, the deaths at calendar-year age $x+1$ include lives whose exact ages at death range from x to $x+2$. There is thus some overlapping of the deaths between adjacent ages, a feature that arises inevitably from the reference of the deaths to the assumed ages at the beginning of the calendar year. This, of course, also applies to the process previously considered in which the living and the deaths were tabulated according to nearest ages at the beginning of the calendar year, so that for the deaths recorded at age x the actual ages at death range from $x-\frac{1}{2}$ to $x+1\frac{1}{2}$. The resulting over-lapping of the deaths between the individual ages suggests that the deaths might be better tabulated according to their actual ages last birthday at death and related to the living at nearest age x at the beginning of the year, but if this were done the deaths at x would not strictly correspond to the living at x. In fact, no subdivision of the lives at the beginning of the year can be made in such a way that the deaths during the ensuing year at age x last birthday exactly correspond. Resort must be had to approximation in one form or another if the deaths are recorded in this way and the possibilities and merits of this process will be discussed later.

3·5. Application of symbols to a calendar-year investigation

The foregoing examples of a calendar-year investigation may be expressed symbolically as follows, measuring t from 1 January of the calendar year of observation:

$$\int_{-\frac{1}{2}}^{\frac{1}{2}} {}_{t}l_{x+r}\,dr = {}_{t}P_{x-\frac{1}{2}}$$

represents the number living at nearest age x at time t so that

$$_{0}P_{x-\frac{1}{2}} = \int_{-\frac{1}{2}}^{\frac{1}{2}} {}_{0}l_{x+r}\,dr$$

is the number living at nearest age x on 1 January.

The notation for the deaths now needs extension. Let $d_{x+r}dr$ represent the deaths in the calendar year among those aged $x+r$ to $x+r+dr$ on 1 January. Then

$$\int_{-\frac{1}{2}}^{\frac{1}{2}} d_{x+r}\,dr = \theta_{(x)}$$

represents the deaths in the calendar year whose nearest age on 1 January was x. We thus have

$$\mathring{q}_x \doteqdot \theta_{(x)}/{}_0P_{x-\frac{1}{2}},$$
$$\mathring{m}_x \doteqdot \theta_{(x)}/({}_0P_{x-\frac{1}{2}} - \tfrac{1}{2}\theta_{(x)}) = \theta_{(x)}/\tfrac{1}{2}({}_0P_{x-\frac{1}{2}} + {}_1P_{x+\frac{1}{2}})$$
$$\doteqdot \theta_{(x)}/({}_0P_{x-\frac{1}{2}} - \theta_{(x)}^{\alpha}),$$

where $\theta_{(x)}^{\alpha}$ represents the number of deaths in $\theta_{(x)}$ which occurred before 1 July.

It should be closely observed that each element $d_{x+r}\,dr$ represents the deaths in the calendar year out of the element ${}_0l_{x+r}\,dr$ living at the start of the year, so that the ratio $d_{x+r}\,dr/{}_0l_{x+r}\,dr$ would represent the observed rate of mortality for the true 'life year' from $x+r$ to $x+r+1$. This is, of course, only a piece of symbolism, because ${}_0l_{x+r}$ is not, in fact, a continuous mathematical function. However, we could take a short interval, such as a week, and define ${}_0l_{x+r}$ as the number living at the beginning of the year whose ages ranged between $x+r$ and $x+r+1$ week, so that d_{x+r} would be the corresponding number of deaths in the ensuing calendar year. Then we could write $\mathring{q}_{x+r} = d_{x+r}/{}_0l_{x+r}$ for the observed mortality rate for the lives aged $x+r$ to $x+r+1$ week at the start of the calendar year. Thus our approximate result

$$\mathring{q}_x \doteqdot \theta_{(x)}/{}_0P_{x-\frac{1}{2}}$$

(=deaths whose nearest age on 1 January was x divided by the population on 1 January at nearest age x) is really a weighted average of all the rates of mortality for all the ages from $x-\frac{1}{2}$ to $x+\frac{1}{2}$. Whether it is a reasonable approximation for the rate of mortality for age x exact depends (1) on whether ${}_0l_{x+r}$ is reasonably constant over the age range $x-\frac{1}{2}$ to $x+\frac{1}{2}$, or, at least, is such that the weighted mean age is close to x, i.e. is such that

$$\int_{-\frac{1}{2}}^{\frac{1}{2}} r\,{}_0l_{x+r}\,dr \bigg/ \int_{-\frac{1}{2}}^{\frac{1}{2}} {}_0l_{x+r}\,dr \doteqdot 0$$

is a reasonably close approximation, and (2) on whether q_{x+r} can be assumed to be approximately linear over the age range $x - \frac{1}{2}$ to $x + \frac{1}{2}$. More generally, apart from random errors included in $\mathring{q}_{x+r}$, it is being assumed that

$$\int_{-\frac{1}{2}}^{\frac{1}{2}} q_{x+r} \, _0l_{x+r} \, dr = q_x \int_{-\frac{1}{2}}^{\frac{1}{2}} \, _0l_{x+r} \, dr.$$

In some special circumstances in which we might know, for example, that there were systematically more lives between ages $x - \frac{1}{2}$ and x than between ages x and $x + \frac{1}{2}$ it might be appropriate to make a sample investigation to estimate the true average age $x - k$ and then treat the ratio of the deaths to the living as giving $\mathring{q}_{x-k}$ instead of $\mathring{q}_x$. This would be an exceptional course to take, but the theoretical point involved should be fully appreciated as the practical processes are always dependent upon the adequacy of the assumptions made.

On 1 January the calendar-year age and the age next birthday are identical, so that the number living at 1 January at calendar-year age x is the same as the number living at age $x - 1$ last birthday, i.e.

$$\int_{-1}^{0} \, _0l_{x+r} \, dr = \, _0P_{x-1}.$$

The deaths at calendar-year age x are the deaths out of all those who were aged $x - 1$ last birthday at the beginning of the year so that

$$\int_{-1}^{0} d_{x+r} \, dr = \theta_{\{x-\frac{1}{2}\}}$$

represents the number of deaths at calendar-year age x.

Thus we have
$$\mathring{q}_{x-\frac{1}{2}} \doteqdot \theta_{\{x-\frac{1}{2}\}} / \, _0P_{x-1},$$
$$\mathring{m}_{x-\frac{1}{2}} \doteqdot \theta_{\{x-\frac{1}{2}\}} / (\, _0P_{x-1} - \tfrac{1}{2}\theta_{\{x-\frac{1}{2}\}})$$
$$\doteqdot \theta_{\{x-\frac{1}{2}\}} / \tfrac{1}{2}(\, _0P_{x-1} + \, _1P_x)$$
$$\doteqdot \theta_{\{x-\frac{1}{2}\}} / (\, _0P_{x-1} - \theta_{\{x-\frac{1}{2}\}}^{\alpha}),$$

where $\theta_{\{x-\frac{1}{2}\}}^{\alpha}$ might represent either the number of deaths included in $\theta_{\{x-\frac{1}{2}\}}$ which occur before 1 July or the number of deaths which occur before their birthdays.

3·6. A policy-year investigation

We now consider the distribution of the living and the corresponding deaths when an investigation is made over a policy year. It is unlikely that this process would be used unless it were desired to analyse the mortality according to duration since entry into insurance, either alone or in conjunction with age. Taking duration alone to begin with, it is apparent that the problem is identical in principle with the distribution over the ages when a life-year investigation is employed because age is simply the duration since birth and life years are similar to policy years if we take birth as equivalent to entry. The whole of what has been said in connexion with a life-year investigation can be interpreted in terms of policy years except that the first policy year (and the last in the case of terminations such as the maturity of endowment policies) may need special treatment. This need not concern us at the present stage, because the present discussion assumes that there are no entrants to the group during the year of observation and no leavers other than by death.

In practice, subdivision by age would usually be required as well as subdivision by duration. Accordingly, the lives reaching their respective policy anniversaries in the first calendar year must be grouped according to age on the policy anniversary. Thus a policy-year investigation involves both the feature of a life-year investigation, that the lives are observed from various points of time in one calendar year to the corresponding points in the next calendar year, and also the feature of a calendar-year investigation, that for any given policy year the lives must be grouped according to age. A particular subgroup would be those lives who were, say, nearest age x at integral duration t in the first calendar year. These lives would be observed over the policy year from exact integral duration t to exact integral duration $t + 1$, and the deaths among them would be counted. In other words, the deaths would be those occurring between the policy anniversaries in the two calendar years, and they would be grouped according to exact duration t and nearest age x, both being determined as on the policy anniversary in the first calendar year. The ratio of deaths to living provides a q-type of rate for duration t for the subgroup of lives whose ages at duration t ranged from $x - \frac{1}{2}$ to $x + \frac{1}{2}$. Assuming that the average age approximates to x the rate may be taken as an approximation to $\mathring{q}_{[x-t]+t}$.

In practice, each policy on the same life may be treated as a separate 'life', and each policy on the same life which is the subject of a claim by death would then be treated as a separate death. Alternatively, steps might be taken to eliminate all duplicates and triplicates, etc., of this kind, in which case some convention would need to be adopted for deciding which policy was to be used for fixing the durations. These complications need not, however, concern us at this stage.

Another possible method would be to tabulate the number of policies in force on 1 January in the second calendar year according to (a) duration on 1 January in completed years (usually referred to as 'curtate duration') and (b) age next birthday at entry plus curtate duration. The deaths would be correspondingly tabulated according to age next birthday at entry and curtate duration. The ratio of the deaths to the in-force for age x next birthday at entry and curtate duration t would provide a central rate applicable to age $x + t$ next birthday and duration t. Assuming, on the average, that the age next birthday is half a year greater than the exact age, this central rate may be taken as approximately equal to $\mathring{m}_{[x-\frac{1}{2}]+t}$.

Further discussion of the complications introduced by the duration factor need not be pursued here because the detailed treatment of 'selection' in mortality investigations is outside the scope of the present volume. It may, however, be mentioned that if a life-year investigation is made, approximations to duration are inevitable just as for a policy-year investigation approximations to age are inevitable. A calendar-year investigation has the distinction that approximations are inevitable both for age and for duration.

3·7. A calendar-year investigation with deaths classified by age at death

So far for a calendar-year investigation we have considered various processes by which the deaths may be classified according to some definition of age on 1 January to correspond with the classification of the living. We now consider the alternative procedure of classifying the deaths according to some definition of age at the date of death (e.g. age last birthday at death) and of attempting to find the corresponding classification for the living on 1 January. It is supposed, of course, that the total deaths exactly correspond to the total living. Without this fundamental overall condition such an attempt would be futile because, in general, we cannot take a group of deaths and find the corresponding living without first defining the living from which the deaths arose. In fact, the principle of correspondence is fundamentally a one-way relation, since the deaths are essentially a subgroup of the living in much the same logical way as the number of 'heads' is a subgroup of the total number of tossings of a given coin. As was mentioned in § 3·4, when the deaths are tabulated according to age last birthday at death there is no way of subdividing the living so that the subgroups of deaths and living would exactly correspond to each other. We are forced to accept an approximation for the correspondence of the subgroups. This is the price that has to be paid for classifying the deaths in exact years of age. It will be remembered that when we classified the living on 1 January and obtained the corresponding deaths we paid the price of mixing up the years of age for the deaths. As F. M. Redington (*J.I.A.* **73**, 209) has pointed out there is involved in this question a kind of uncertainty principle: exact correspondence means vagueness in the years of age for the deaths; exact years of age for the deaths means vagueness in the degree of correspondence for the subgroups. In both cases the individual values of q or m may have little meaning in themselves. It is by virtue of the total correspondence condition that meaning is given to the *set* of values of q or m. A sound process of graduation, in suitable conditions and on certain assumptions, is an operation on the set of values which, as will be seen later, extracts from the figures their underlying meaning in terms of rates for individual ages.

3·8. Classification of the living in half-year age-ranges

We will now consider possible ways of classifying the living so that the subgroups approximately correspond when the deaths are tabulated according to age last birthday at death. We could, as a first approximation, relate the deaths at age x last birthday to the living on 1 January at nearest age x. But some of the deaths at age x last birthday may have been in the age-range $x-1$ to $x-\frac{1}{2}$ on 1 January (i.e. included in the subgroup for nearest age $x-1$) and some may have been in the age-range $x+\frac{1}{2}$ to $x+1$ on 1 January (i.e. included in the subgroup for nearest age $x+1$). On the other hand, some of the lives at nearest age x on 1 January may have died during the calendar year of experience at age last birthday $x-1$ or $x+1$.

TABLE 3·1

Subgroup of the living on 1 January	Years of age and fractions of the year for which the lives are exposed on the average		
	$x-1$ to x	x to $x+1$	$x+1$ to $x+2$
P_1	$\frac{3}{4}$	$\frac{1}{4}$	—
P_2	$\frac{1}{4}$	$\frac{3}{4}$	—
P_3	—	$\frac{3}{4}$	$\frac{1}{4}$
P_4	—	$\frac{1}{4}$	$\frac{3}{4}$

These overlaps suggest that the living might be better tabulated in half-year age-ranges. To consider this possibility let P_1, P_2, P_3 and P_4 represent the numbers living in the age-ranges $x-1$ to $x-\frac{1}{2}$, $x-\frac{1}{2}$ to x, x to $x+\frac{1}{2}$ and $x+\frac{1}{2}$ to $x+1$ respectively. Then, assuming a uniform distribution of fractional ages within each subgroup, P_1 are exposed to the risk of death in the first half of the year of age x to $x+1$ but in the second half of the calendar year, and the exposure is for a quarter of a year on the average, because those aged a day or two over $x-1$ are exposed for only a day or two and those aged nearly $x-\frac{1}{2}$ are exposed for nearly half a year.* Similarly, P_4 are exposed in the second half of the year of age x to $x+1$ in the first half of the calendar year for a quarter of a year on the average. P_2 and P_3 are each exposed, on the average, for three-quarters of a year in the year of age x to $x+1$ in the calendar year. The balance of the year's exposure in each case applies to adjacent ages. Thus the exposure is allocated on the average as shown in Table 3·1. The approximate exposed-to-risk corresponding to the deaths at age x last birthday is therefore

$$\tfrac{1}{4}P_1+\tfrac{3}{4}P_2+\tfrac{3}{4}P_3+\tfrac{1}{4}P_4.$$

* In calculating the average exposure any life dying is deemed to be exposed up to the $(x+1)$th birthday or 31 December, whichever is the first to occur.

It will be observed that, provided the values of P are not greatly dissimilar, the fractions of a year of exposure show a reasonable balance between the first and second halves of the year of age and between the first and second halves of the calendar year. It is not, in general, unreasonable to regard n lives aged x on 1 January and exposed from 1 January until 30 June and n different (but similar) lives aged $x + \frac{1}{2}$ on 1 July and exposed from 1 July to 31 December as equivalent to n lives aged x on 1 January and exposed throughout the whole year. In practice, it is not usually worth while to pursue such niceties of balance, and it is usually sufficient, particularly when allowance is made for new entrants and leavers, to add the various fractions of a year of 'risk-time' in the relevant year of age even if the total 'risk-time' is not uniformly spread over the year of age or over the period of experience, provided that the fractions of risk are allocated to the right years of age and the total of the fractions allocated is equal to the total exposure to a sufficient degree of approximation.

The idea of 'risk-time' could be applied with greater precision by allocating to each life aged exactly $x + r$ on 1 January its exact fraction $1 - r$ of 'risk-time' in the calendar year in the year of age x to $x + 1$, so that the total exposure in that year of age would be

$$\int_0^1 (1 - r)({}_0l_{x-r} + {}_0l_{x+r})\,dr.$$

If this were done there would be a strict correspondence between the deaths and the risk-time, but there would still be vagueness in the definition of the resulting rates and the ages to which they apply.

3·9. Classification of the living according to age last birthday

In practice, it is unusual to go to the length of classifying the living in half-year age-ranges. Since the only lives who could die at age x last birthday in the calendar year are those who were aged $x - 1$ or x last birthday on 1 January, a classification of the living according to age last birthday would be a reasonable procedure. On the usual uniformity assumption, those aged $x - 1$ last birthday on 1 January are exposed for half a year on the average in the calendar year in the year of age x to $x + 1$. Similarly, those aged x

last birthday on 1 January are exposed for half a year on the average. The approximate exposed-to-risk corresponding to the deaths at age x last birthday would then be half the numbers living at age $x-1$ and at age x last birthday on 1 January.

3·10. Classification of the living according to nearest ages

If the living were classified according to nearest age on 1 January we might substitute one-eighth of the numbers living at nearest ages $x-1$ and $x+1$ for $\frac{1}{4}(P_1+P_4)$ in the formula

$$\tfrac{1}{4}P_1+\tfrac{3}{4}P_2+\tfrac{3}{4}P_3+\tfrac{1}{4}P_4,$$

if it were reasonable to assume that the living between ages $x-1\frac{1}{2}$ and $x-1$ were approximately equal in number to those between ages $x-1$ and $x-\frac{1}{2}$ and similarly for the two parts of the living at nearest age $x+1$. It is, however, questionable whether it is better to approximate by bringing in some living who could not possibly die in the year of age rather than to approximate by leaving out some who could, as is done by using the unadjusted number living at nearest age x as the exposed-to-risk corresponding to the deaths at age x last birthday. In practice, both approximations depend on the assumption that the numbers living at adjacent ages are not greatly dissimilar (or are approximately linear in x), and if this assumption is justified the results by the two methods cannot be significantly different.

Instead of trying to bring the living as closely as possible into line with the deaths, the deaths could be redistributed to bring them more into line with the living at nearest age x. By exactly similar considerations as apply to the redistribution of the living, one-eighth of the number of deaths at age x last birthday can be associated with the living at nearest age $x-1$ and one-eighth at $x+1$. Thus the redistributed deaths corresponding more closely to the living at nearest age x would be $\tfrac{1}{8}\theta_{x-1}+\tfrac{3}{4}\theta_x+\tfrac{1}{8}\theta_{x+1}$. A closer association could be achieved by subdividing the deaths into half-year age-ranges in the same way as was done for the living. The number of deaths approximately corresponding to the living at nearest age x would then be $\tfrac{1}{4}\theta_1+\tfrac{3}{4}\theta_2+\tfrac{3}{4}\theta_3+\tfrac{1}{4}\theta_4$, where θ_1, etc., were the numbers of deaths in the four half-year age-ranges from $x-\frac{1}{2}$ to $x+\frac{3}{2}$. This process achieves a higher degree of correspondence at the expense of precision in the definition of the ages to which the resulting rates apply. By adjusting the deaths we are really attempting to make a closer approach to the mortality rate for the subgroup of lives at age x nearest on 1 January. Owing, however, to the relatively large differences between the numbers of deaths at adjacent ages that can occur in a small experience, the averaging process is much more hazardous when performed on the deaths than when performed on the living. The individual rates become even more meaningless, although as a set the rates would, of course, be acceptable.

If a redistribution is to be made it is usually preferable to operate on the living rather than on the deaths, because, as has already been mentioned, errors in the living have less effect on the mortality rate than errors in the deaths. In practice, however, it is usually unnecessary to make such meticulous redistributions at all, but care needs to be exercised when the deaths and the living do not exactly correspond if there is a sharp break in the run of the numbers recorded at successive ages. An important example of this disturbing circumstance is often found in pension-fund data where an option to retire at, say, exact age 60 may mean a sudden drop in the numbers at age 60 compared with those at ages 58 and 59. Special treatment is required to cope with difficulties of this kind.

3·11. Deaths tabulated according to duration at death

A further complication of the problem of distributing the living to correspond with the deaths, or vice versa, may sometimes arise if ages are determined by reference to age at entry and duration. For example, the deaths in a calendar-year experience of assured lives might be tabulated according to age next birthday at entry x and curtate duration t at the date of death. The living on the valuation date, 1 January, might be similarly tabulated according to age next birthday at entry x and curtate duration t on 1 January. Clearly so far as age at entry is concerned there is strict correspondence, but for the durations there is a problem of securing approximate correspondence. The deaths at x and t could come from the living at x and $t-1$ or from the living at x and t. This at once suggests, on the usual uniformity assumption, that we could

3

either average the numbers living at durations t and $t-1$ and associate the result with the deaths at duration t, or average the numbers of deaths at durations t and $t+1$ and associate the result with the living at duration t. In the former case the resulting rate would approximate to $\mathring{q}_{(x-\frac{1}{2})+t}$; in the latter case it would approximate to $\mathring{q}_{(x-\frac{1}{2})+t+\frac{1}{2}}$. If age-rates, without distinction with regard to duration, were required, the numerators and denominators would be aggregated for all subgroups with a common value of $x+t$, remembering that, on the usual uniformity assumption, age x next birthday plus curtate duration t is, on the average, attained age $x+t$, with a range from $x+t-1$ to $x+t+1$.

3·12. Central rates

Whatever methods are used for classifying the living the appropriate course for central rates would be to deduct one-half of the number of deaths at age x last birthday (or at assumed age x) from the number assumed to be living at integral age x on 1 January (e.g. the unadjusted or adjusted number at nearest age x). The result would provide a suitable denominator to be applied to the number of deaths at age x last birthday to obtain the central rate at age x. It is, of course, still assumed that there are no new entrants or leavers. Alternatively, a census of the living on 1 July according to ages last birthday would provide suitable denominators. Since the lives aged x last birthday at 1 July are the survivors of those living at nearest age x on 1 January there is an obvious link with the method of obtaining $\mathring{q}_x$ from the deaths at age x last birthday and the living on 1 January at age x nearest. Similarly, since the living on 1 July at age x last birthday provides an approximation to the mean population at age x last birthday throughout the year, there is an obvious link with the 'census method' discussed later in the chapter.

3·13. Total deaths and total exposure

Whatever methods are used for allocating the living and the deaths over the ages the procedure must ensure that all the living and all the deaths are so allocated. For example, each individual death should be included in the numerator of one and only one mortality rate or one-half may be allocated to each of two adjacent ages. In certain special cases other complementary fractions may be appropriate; for example, an eighth may be allocated to one age, three-quarters to the next age and the remaining eighth to the next. Similarly, each individual among the living must be included in one and only one denominator for the mortality rates; or each individual may be suitably distributed in complementary fractions over two or more adjacent ages. The essential principle is that in distributing the deaths and the living over the ages (and durations) the total number of deaths and the total exposure must be exactly reproduced.

3·14. Methods based on ages last birthday at death expressed in symbols

The use of ages last birthday at death in an experience over a calendar year with an approximate association of the living over the successive ages may be expressed in symbols as follows:

As before, we have for the living on 1 January at nearest age x

$$\int_{-\frac{1}{2}}^{\frac{1}{2}} {}_0 l_{x+r}\, dr = {}_0 P_{x-\frac{1}{2}}.$$

The mean between the populations at ages $x-1$ and x last birthday on 1 January is $\frac{1}{2}({}_0P_{x-1}+{}_0P_x)$. We thus have

$$\mathring{q}_x \doteqdot \theta_x/{}_0P_{x-\frac{1}{2}}$$
$$\doteqdot \theta_x/\tfrac{1}{2}({}_0P_x+{}_0P_{x-1})$$
$$\doteqdot \theta_x/(\tfrac{1}{8}{}_0P_{x-\frac{3}{2}}+\tfrac{3}{4}{}_0P_{x-\frac{1}{2}}+\tfrac{1}{8}{}_0P_{x+\frac{1}{2}})$$
$$\doteqdot (\tfrac{1}{8}\theta_{x-1}+\tfrac{3}{4}\theta_x+\tfrac{1}{8}\theta_{x+1})/{}_0P_{x-\frac{1}{2}},$$
$$\mathring{m}_x \doteqdot \theta_x/{}_{\frac{1}{2}}P_x$$
$$\doteqdot \theta_x/({}_0P_{x-\frac{1}{2}}-\tfrac{1}{2}\theta_x)$$
$$\doteqdot \theta_x/({}_0P_{x-\frac{1}{2}}-\theta_x^{\alpha}),$$

where θ_x^{α} represents the deaths at age x last birthday in the first half of the calendar year.

3·15. The 'census method'

In connexion with the central rate, approximations have already been made several times to the 'mean population at age x last birthday throughout the year'; for example, the number starting the year at nearest age x less half the number of deaths (§3·4) or a census total on 1 July at age x last birthday (§3·4) or the mean between the number living at nearest age x on 1 January and the number living at nearest age $(x+1)$ at the end of the year (§3·5). Moreover, the notion of the 'mean population' as the denominator for the central rate has not been confined to a calendar-year investigation. Further, if we have an approximation to the mean population we can obtain a suitable exposed-to-risk for the q-type of rate by adding half the number of deaths to the mean population, thus approximating to the relevant number starting the year.

There is, however, one method of approximating to the mean population in a calendar-year investigation (particularly in life-office investigations) that is generally treated in the literature as an entirely distinct method under the special name of the 'census method'.

In actual fact, when censuses at yearly intervals are used the method is not significantly different from the methods already described. The particular method arose from an analogy with the process used for obtaining rates of mortality from the national decennial censuses and the deaths in the intervening years. A mean population at age x last birthday over the 10-year period was obtained from the two census figures for age x last birthday. The last time this method was used for the national statistics was after the 1911 census when the English Life Tables No. 7 were constructed from the 1901 and 1911 censuses and the deaths for the years 1901–10. Since then the method used has been to treat the census figures as suitable approximations for the mean populations for the 3-year period centred on the census year, the slight discrepancy between the census date and 1 July of the middle year of the 3-year period being usually ignored.

This more modern process would be inconvenient for life-office work because a census on 1 July is not usually available. On the other hand, offices usually make up their valuation totals, which are essentially in the form of censuses of the policies in force, as on 31 December of each year. If these statistics include the numbers (of policies) at age x last birthday at the beginning and end of the calendar year (i.e. $_0P_x$ and $_1P_x$) the mean between these two numbers would be an approximation to the mean population at age x last birthday and would provide a suitable denominator to apply to the number of deaths (death-claims) in the calendar year at age x last birthday in order to obtain $\mathring{m}_x$. It should be particularly noted that we are here averaging the numbers at the beginning and end of the year *at the same age*. Hitherto, when we have used the numbers at the beginning and end of the year we have averaged $_0P_{x-\frac{1}{2}}$ and $_1P_{x+\frac{1}{2}}$ (i.e. the survivors out of $_0P_{x-\frac{1}{2}}$) for $\mathring{m}_x$ or $_0P_{x-1}$ and $_1P_x$ for $\mathring{m}_{x-\frac{1}{2}}$. The population at age x last birthday at time t is $_tP_x = \int_0^1 {}_tl_{x+r}dr$, and the mean population at age x last birthday throughout the year is thus

$$\int_0^1 {}_tP_x\,dt = \int_0^1 \int_0^1 {}_tl_{x+r}\,dr\,dt,$$

and we may evidently use $\frac{1}{2}({}_0P_x + {}_1P_x)$ as an approximation to the mean population provided that $_tP_x$ is approximately linear in t. The rates of mortality at age x by the 'census method' are thus

$$\mathring{q}_x \doteqdot \theta_x / \tfrac{1}{2}({}_0P_x + {}_1P_x + \theta_x),$$
$$\mathring{m}_x \doteqdot \theta_x / \tfrac{1}{2}({}_0P_x + {}_1P_x).$$

In practice, life offices usually group their policies on 31 December of each year according to nearest integral ages or according to some other definition of age which approximates, on the average, to integral ages, e.g. according to age next birthday at entry plus curtate duration of the policy. Evidently, if the censuses are according to nearest age the above 'census-method' formulae can be used if we substitute throughout $x - \frac{1}{2}$ for x, both for the populations and for the deaths, and interpret $x - \frac{1}{2}$ 'last birthday' as meaning 'aged between $x - \frac{1}{2}$ and $x + \frac{1}{2}$' in the same way as age x last birthday means 'aged between x and $x + 1$'. Thus $_0P_{x-\frac{1}{2}}$ can be interpreted as the number living on 1 January (or the previous 31 December) either at age $x - \frac{1}{2}$ 'last birthday' or at age x nearest birthday. Similarly, $\theta_{x-\frac{1}{2}}$ represents the number of deaths in the year whose age at death was $x-\frac{1}{2}$ 'last birthday' or x nearest birthday. Thus, if the ages are nearest birthday throughout, the 'census method' provides values of $\mathring{q}_{x-\frac{1}{2}}$ and $\mathring{m}_{x-\frac{1}{2}}$.

If the valuation statistics are compiled according to some other approximation to integral ages the 'census method' can still be used to obtain rates for half-ages provided that the deaths are similarly classified according to some form of approximation to age $x-\frac{1}{2}$ 'last birthday'.

When we come in Chapter 5 to discuss the adjustments for new entrants and leavers we shall see that the 'census method' has the merit of automatically making an approximate allowance for these disturbances on the basis of giving half a year's exposure only to each new entrant and leaver during the calendar year.

It now remains to show that the census method is only one way of applying the usual principles. This is simply done by using the identity $_1P_x = {}_0P_{x-1} - \theta_{(x-\frac{1}{2})}$, that is, the population aged x last birthday at the end of the year is equal to the population aged $x-1$ last birthday at the beginning of the year minus the deaths during the year whose ages last birthday at the beginning of the year were $x-1$.

The census formulae for $\mathring{q}$ and $\mathring{m}$ can now be rewritten as follows:

$$\mathring{q}_x \doteqdot \theta_x / \tfrac{1}{2} \left({}_0P_x + {}_0P_{x-1} - \theta_{(x-\frac{1}{2})} + \theta_x \right),$$
$$\mathring{m}_x \doteqdot \theta_x / \tfrac{1}{2} \left({}_0P_x + {}_0P_{x-1} - \theta_{(x-\frac{1}{2})} \right).$$

$\theta_{(x-\frac{1}{2})}$ and θ_x are, of course, approximately equal and small relatively to P. If this were not so the averaging processes used in the various formulae would break down. Accordingly, $\theta_{(x-\frac{1}{2})}$ and θ_x can each be taken as an approximation for the other in the denominator of $\mathring{q}$ and $\mathring{m}$. Thus if we substitute θ_x for $\theta_{(x-\frac{1}{2})}$ in the denominator of $\mathring{q}$ we have

$$\mathring{q}_x \doteqdot \theta_x / \tfrac{1}{2} \left({}_0P_x + {}_0P_{x-1} \right)$$
$$\doteqdot \theta_x / {}_0P_{x-\frac{1}{2}},$$

which are both in the usual form of the ratio of the number of deaths to the number living at the beginning of the year.

By substituting θ_x for $\theta_{(x-\frac{1}{2})}$ in the denominator of $\mathring{m}$ we similarly obtain $\mathring{m}$ in the usual form

$$\mathring{m}_x \doteqdot \theta_x / \tfrac{1}{2} \left({}_0P_x + {}_0P_{x-1} - \theta_x \right)$$
$$\doteqdot \theta_x / \left({}_0P_{x-\frac{1}{2}} - \tfrac{1}{2}\theta_x \right).$$

It will be seen in later chapters that this reduction of the census method to the ordinary form is still possible when allowance is made for new entrants and leavers and when duration is taken into account as well as age. In the meantime, it is a useful exercise for the reader to consider the modifications possible in the applications of the various methods of using deaths at age x last birthday, including the census method, if the numbers of deaths are subdivided into their α and β parts, i.e. death before and after the birthday in the calendar year of death.

3·16. Classification of methods

From time to time attempts have been made to classify the various procedures that have been used for mortality investigations. In this book the development of life-year, calendar-year and policy-year investigations in successive stages may have given the appearance of a classification of method into these three classes, but it has become apparent that within each of these procedures there are important differences of method according to the way in which the data of the living and deaths are tabulated or used. This has been discussed in detail for a calendar-year investigation, partly because this lends itself readily to exposition and partly because of the obvious importance of calendar-year investigations in practical work.

In the literature of the subject and in actuarial students' training courses from time to time different meanings have been attached to the three phrases, 'life-year method', 'calendar-year method' and 'policy-year method', and it is desirable to elucidate these different uses of the phrases so that there may be no confusion between our own and other forms of development. We have not used the labels 'life-year', 'calendar-year' and 'policy-year' attached to the word 'method', but we have found it necessary to attach them, with quite specific and fully defined meanings, to the word 'investigation'. Originally, mortality investigations were based on the principle that the lives should be 'followed through' their years of life from birthday to birthday. Then when it was realized that mortality varies with duration since entry into assurance, methods of investigation directed to measuring 'selection' were devised and the principle that the policies should be 'followed through' their years of life from policy anniversary to policy anniversary was a natural development. However, for many practical problems in life assurance, friendly society and other actuarial work, data concerning the living (or the in-force) and the deaths (or death-claims) were often readily available in calendar years. This was, of course, because the calendar year was commonly used for accounting purposes and because the ends of accounting years are naturally chosen as the dates for actuarial valuations of the liabilities and assets. The third process of following the lives, or policies, through successive calendar years was thus a development out of practical circumstances.

It was natural, therefore, to regard the type of method used in any particular case, and the particular label to be applied to it, as being determined by whether the experience started and ended on the birthdays or on the policy anniversaries or on some fixed date (e.g. 1 January) in given calendar years. This method of classifying the various methods in use was not affected by the inclusion in some investigations of an allowance on an approximate basis for the fractional period of exposure before the birthday in the first calendar year in the case of a life-year investigation or of a corresponding allowance for the period before the first policy anniversary in the first calendar year in the case of a policy-year investigation. It was natural to associate the different processes with the way in which the ages were fixed, which might be on an exact basis from birthday to birthday, or by grouping according to nearest integral ages on policy anniversaries, or by grouping according to ages last birthday on 1 January of successive calendar years or in some other way.

In 1894 W. J. H. Whittall (*J.I.A.* **31**, 161) pointed out that the idea of following the lives through various kinds of years was vague, and he claimed that what was in question was the way in which the rates of mortality were followed through various kinds of year and that the vital point was the way in which the ages at death were determined. He made the further point that the allocation of the deaths to the proper ages is more important than complete precision in fixing the exposed-to-risk. This is, of course, quite true from a purely arithmetical point of view, looking at each mortality rate separately, since a given error in the small numerator of the rate of mortality is of much greater significance than a similar error in the large denominator. Whittall concluded that the significant feature determining whether a given method was a life-year, policy-year or calendar-year method should be the way in which the ages at death are fixed. Are they the ages last birthday, or are they the assumed ages on the last policy anniversary or are they the assumed ages on 1 January of the calendar year of death? Thus the process of obtaining rates of mortality from an investigation over a calendar year with deaths tabulated according to age last birthday at death (and used unadjusted in this form) would be called 'a life-year method' because, despite the fact that the total deaths are those occurring in a calendar year, the deaths are classified in strict years of age with the exposed-to-risk approximately corresponding.

If the numbers of deaths were adjusted to correspond approximately to a classification of the living according to nearest age on 1 January, the process would be called 'a calendar-year method'. If the deaths at age x last birthday are related to the living on 1 January at nearest age x, we could presumably regard the process either as a life-year method with the living approximately corresponding to the deaths or as a calendar-year method with the deaths approximately corresponding to the living. In fact, as soon as approximation is allowed in the correspondence relation any system of classification of method becomes ambiguous. If the correspondence relation is strictly ensured then the classification should be identical whether attention is focused on the way in which the living are classified (with the deaths corresponding) or on the way in which the deaths are classified (with the living corresponding). But if the deaths at nearest age x on 1 January are associated with the living at nearest age x on 1 January, it is possible to regard the resulting rate as an average rate for the lives aged $x+r$ on 1 January over their life-years $x+r$ to $x+r+1$ for all values of r from $-\frac{1}{2}$ to $\frac{1}{2}$. For these reasons we have avoided the use of any system of classification of this kind, preferring to describe as precisely as we can the processes employed without attaching labels to them.

Methods involving only approximate correspondence are often used in practice because they represent a saving in effort and expense without significant loss of accuracy for the purpose in view. Such a method yields a set of mortality rates from the total experience—individual rates may have little or no significance in isolation—which are used either for comparison with a set of rates from a standard table, balancing together divergencies of opposite sign, or as a basis for producing a new set of graduated rates. A condition of success in using methods involving only approximate correspondence is the avoidance of bias of any kind in balancing one group with another when approximating to ages or average periods of exposure. This need to avoid bias applies also to age approximations even when correspondence is strictly preserved.

3·17. Graphical representation of a single calendar year's experience

It may be helpful to some students to express in graphical form the various processes of distributing over the individual ages the total exposed-to-risk and deaths for a single calendar-year's experience. For this purpose it is again assumed that there are no new entrants or leavers during the year of observation. There are two variables, age and time. The age variable r is measured from an age origin x; the time variable t is measured from the beginning of the calendar year, so that $t = 1$ represents the end of the year of observation. In Fig. 3·1, t is measured along the horizontal axis and r is measured along the vertical axis. If we now choose a small finite interval of *age* (e.g. 1 week), we can imagine erected off the plane of the paper on the r-axis a histogram representing the distribution at time 0 of the living between age $x+r$ and age $x+r+1$ week for each value of r by steps of 1 week. If we also choose a similar interval of *time*—it is convenient to choose the same interval of 1 week as for age, although it is not essential that it should be the same—we can imagine a set of histograms at time intervals of 1 week such that they represent the survivors at weekly intervals of the original population at time 0 as the population progresses through time. A given group of lives aged $x+r$ to $x+r+1$ week at time 0 can then be followed along a diagonal strip of squares of side 1 week at an angle of 45° to the two axes. Vertical distributions show the age distribution at a given point of time; horizontal distributions show the numbers reaching a given age as time passes; consecutive human life follows the diagonal lines. It is thus only on diagonal lines that complete 'correspondence' applies between the living and the deaths.

Fig. 3·2 represents the deaths, with time and age similarly measured along the horizontal and vertical axes respectively.

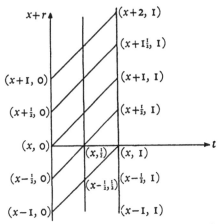

Fig. 3·1. Plan of the distribution of the living at successive ages at successive points of time.

We now imagine erected off the plane of the paper on each vertical set of squares of side 1 week a histogram representing the age distribution (age at death) of the deaths in the particular week of the calendar year to which the vertical set of squares relates. Similarly, each horizontal set of squares represents the time distribution of the deaths in the calendar year in the particular week of age (at death) to which the horizontal set of squares relates. The corresponding diagonal histograms represent the time *and* age-at-death distribution of the deaths in the calendar year that are in strict correspondence with the living in the particular week of age at the beginning of the calendar year to which the diagonal set of squares relates; thus the 'commencing' age remains constant for each diagonal histogram. The situation could be notionally 'idealized' by thinking of the population at the beginning of the year as being indefinitely great, by reducing indefinitely the small age and time intervals and by 'transcending' the fact that deaths occur in 'unit packets'. Then we could think of all the histograms (vertical, horizontal and diagonal) as becoming frequency curves and Figs. 3·1 and 3·2 becoming frequency surfaces. Then each diagonal curve of Fig. 3·1 would represent a section of an l-curve from age $x+r$ to age $x+r+1$, through the period of one calendar year. Similarly, the corresponding diagonal curve of Fig. 3·2 would

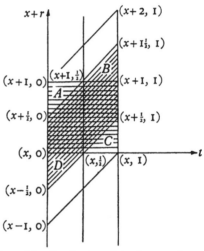

Fig. 3·2. Plan of the distribution of deaths at various ages in successive small intervals of time.

represent a section of a death-curve (μl) from age $x+r$ to age $x+r+1$ and over the same period of one calendar year. The separate diagonal curves would not be related to each other in any real way because they would represent the partial life histories of different groups of lives commencing the calendar year. We could, however, think of them as being related in a statistical sense because the individual groups of lives represent the age distribution at the successive points of time throughout the year of the whole group of lives forming the basis of the investigation. It is, in fact, only because there may be, in this sense and to a sufficient degree, an approximate relationship (albeit with fluctuations) between the numbers in the respective subgroups that certain approximate processes are sufficiently accurate for practical purposes.

Returning to consideration of Fig. 3·2, the area shaded diagonally represents the bases of the segments of the various histograms which comprise the total deaths in the calendar year out of the living at the beginning of the year at nearest age x; the segments of the histograms covering the area shaded horizontally represent all the deaths in the calendar year at age x last birthday at death; and there is a large common area shaded both horizontally and diagonally. It will be seen that there is no group of lives at 1 January which can be

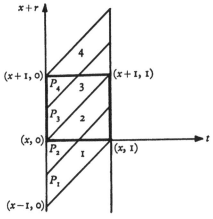

Fig. 3·3. Risk-time corresponding to half-yearly age-ranges of the living at the beginning of the year.

defined so that the horizontally shaded area precisely corresponds. We can regard the process of relating the deaths at age x last birthday to the living at nearest age x as an approximation to the mortality rate for the lives aged x nearest (and hence an approximation to $\mathring{q}_x$) by means of a substitution of the deaths corresponding to the horizontally shaded area for those corresponding to the diagonally shaded area. That is, we are substituting the deaths corresponding to the triangles marked A and C in Fig. 3·2 for those corresponding to B and D respectively. As we remarked in §3·8 there is a fair enough exchange as a whole both as regards parts of the calendar year and parts of the year of age.

We can now show graphically how it is that the expression $(\frac{1}{4}P_1+\frac{3}{4}P_2+\frac{3}{4}P_3+\frac{1}{4}P_4)$, considered in §3·8, is likely to provide a closer approximation than (P_2+P_3) to the risk-time corresponding to the deaths at age x last birthday. In Fig. 3·3 the four parallelograms marked 1, 2, 3 and 4 correspond to the risk-time arising from P_1, P_2, P_3 and P_4 respectively for the q-type of rate. The corresponding risk-time for the m-type of rate would, of course, be the histogram segments for the living erected on the respective parallelograms.

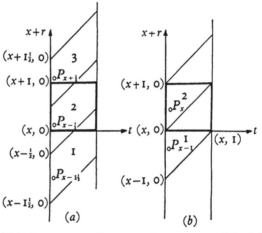

Fig. 3·4. Risk-time corresponding to yearly age-ranges of the living at the beginning of the year (a) nearest integral ages, (b) ages last birthday.

It will be seen from Fig. 3·3 that only a quarter of each of the parallelograms 1 and 4 lie within the square bounded by the thick lines. This square corresponds to the deaths in the calendar year at age x last birthday. On the other hand, three-quarters of each of the parallelograms 2 and 3 lie within this square. Thus by using the expression $(\frac{1}{4}P_1+\frac{3}{4}P_2+\frac{3}{4}P_3+\frac{1}{4}P_4)$ instead of (P_2+P_3) we reduce the effect of serious divergencies between the numbers living in the successive half-year age-ranges and we also confine the deaths and the exposure more closely to the year of age x to $x+1$. But the approximation still depends on the numbers within each half-year age-range being reasonably well spread over such half-year.

Fig. 3·4 shows the corresponding position when the living are

tabulated in the yearly age-ranges (a) according to nearest integral
ages and (b) according to ages last birthday.

In (a) one-eighth of each of the parallelograms 1 and 3 lie within
the heavily lined square, while three-quarters of parallelogram 2
lies within the square. This checks the formula given in §3·10 in
terms of the living at nearest ages $x - 1$, x and $x + 1$. It is, however,
a moot point whether this formula really achieves any improvement
over the simple process of taking $_0P_{x-\frac{1}{2}}$ as the exposed-to-risk corresponding to θ_x. By using the living at nearest age x unadjusted we
exclude altogether some lives who could die in the relevant year of
age and calendar year, and we include too much exposure for those
aged x nearest, that is, we exclude the approximate exposure of
one-quarter of a year for those between $x - 1$ and $x - \frac{1}{2}$ and those
aged between $x + \frac{1}{2}$ and $x + 1$ (i.e. two half-ages) and include an
extra one-quarter of a year for those aged between $x - \frac{1}{2}$ and $x + \frac{1}{2}$
as an approximate substitute; these lives being exposed on their
own account on a broad approximation for three-quarters of a year,
on the average.

On the other hand, by including an adjustment for the living at
nearest ages $x - 1$ and $x + 1$ we include some lives who could not
possibly die in the year of age x to $x + 1$ in the calendar year of the
investigation. The use of the fraction one-eighth is based on the
broad approximation that those at the beginning of the year aged
less than $x - 1$ exact and more than $x + 1$ are not exposed at all and
those aged between $x - 1$ and $x - \frac{1}{2}$ and between $x + \frac{1}{2}$ and $x + 1$ are
exposed, on the average, for a quarter of a year in the relevant year
of age and calendar year.

In Fig. 3·4 (b) one-half of each of the parallelograms 1 and 2 lie
within the heavily lined square corresponding to the deaths at
age x last birthday in the calendar year, and this is the justification
for the formula $\frac{1}{2}(_0P_{x-1} + _0P_x)$ given in §3·14 as an approximation
to the exposed-to-risk corresponding to θ_x when the living are
tabulated according to ages last birthday.

Clearly, the relative success of these various processes as approximations to the 'risk-time' depends on the distribution of the living
over the age-ranges brought into account. If there is a fairly uniform
distribution or if there is a reasonably regular linear progression the

various processes produce closely similar results. If this is not so, no general statement about their relative accuracy can be made. In practice, refinements in procedure are often not worth while, particularly when approximate allowance has to be made for new entrants and leavers and when the needs of the practical situation and the purpose to be served by the investigation are brought into consideration. Broad approximations are then seen to be adequate and meticulous adjustments are out of place. It is, however, necessary to appreciate the underlying principles if only so that major errors and biased processes may be avoided. When several years of experience are combined together and many of the lives remain in the investigation for a number of years, the usual approximate procedures practically always result in the exposure being necessarily allocated to the correct years of age, except possibly for the first and last years of exposure of individual lives. In such circumstances there is often an advantage in allocating the deaths to their correct years of age rather than to strive after as complete a correspondence as possible at the price either of tabulating the deaths to conform to the ages of the living at the commencement of years of exposure or of re-allocating them to conform approximately to this position. In practice, however, even this advantage is not to be regarded very seriously.

CHAPTER 4

COMBINATION OF TWO OR MORE YEARS OF EXPERIENCE

4·1. The reasons for combining several years of experience

It is obvious that if we want to combine the experience of two or more years (life, calendar or policy years) and obtain combined mortality rates for the whole period the straightforward way of doing this would be to tabulate the exposed-to-risk and deaths for each year separately and combine the results. Indeed, the process would be exactly the same as if we had taken out the experience for two groups of lives for the same year of experience and then combined the results into a single experience. The two groups might well exhibit different mortality rates, in which case the combined experience would be a weighted average of the two experiences, the weights, of course, differing for each age. If the mortality of a single group is changing as the years go by, as has in fact been the general experience for the past couple of centuries, the combination of two or more years of experience involves exactly the same idea of a weighted average of the separate experiences, with the weights varying with the age.

Owing to the seasonal variation and the observed fact that, apart from the general trend, some years show worse mortality than others, the combination of the experiences of a short period of years may be a desirable procedure to obtain a set of mortality rates showing the current average level of mortality. For extensive experiences, however, it is nowadays fairly common practice to record the rates for individual years (usually calendar years) and to make the combination in the final stages. For smaller experiences, particularly those arising in the day-to-day work of an actuary, a combined experience for a period of years may be desirable to provide an adequate volume of data and to reduce the large fluctuations from year to year due to smallness of numbers. The experience over a quinquennium between two valuation dates is often a

H & P

practical requirement as a part of the investigation of the experience of a friendly society or pension fund prior to fixing the basis for a valuation of the fund.

There are available short-cut techniques for the combined experience of a period of years that have long been part of the actuary's tool-kit, and it is necessary now to indicate the principles involved in these techniques. For the time being we shall continue to assume that there are no new entrants or leavers, and this assumption will be extended to apply over the whole period of the combined experience.

4·2. Combination of two or more years' experience

The exposition of the process of combining the experience of two or more years will be simplified by writing $_0P_{\{x\}}$, $_1P_{\{x\}}$, $_2P_{\{x\}}$, etc., for the living at age x at the beginning of the successive years of experience and by writing $_0\theta_{\{x\}}$, $_1\theta_{\{x\}}$, $_2\theta_{\{x\}}$, etc., for the corresponding deaths at age x in the successive years. The x in $_tP_{\{x\}}$ is intended to represent integral ages and may be nearest ages so that $_tP_{\{x\}} = {}_tP_{x-\frac{1}{2}}$. Similarly, $_t\theta_{\{x\}}$ represents the deaths in the year whose ages were x at the beginning of the year (e.g. x nearest at the beginning of the year). Then we have

$$_0\mathring{q}_x \doteqdot {}_0\theta_{\{x\}}/_0P_{\{x\}},$$

$$_1\mathring{q}_x \doteqdot {}_1\theta_{\{x\}}/_1P_{\{x\}}.$$

The combined rate for the two years is therefore

$$\mathring{q}_x \doteqdot ({}_0\theta_{\{x\}} + {}_1\theta_{\{x\}})/({}_0P_{\{x\}} + {}_1P_{\{x\}}),$$

and generally for n years

$$\mathring{q}_x \doteqdot \sum_{t=0}^{n-1} {}_t\theta_{\{x\}} \Big/ \sum_{t=0}^{n-1} {}_tP_{\{x\}}.$$

In a 2-year period if $_0P_{\{x\}}$ and $_1P_{\{x\}}$ are approximately equal the set of values of $\mathring{q}_x$ would be approximately equal to the set of values of $\frac{1}{2}({}_0\mathring{q}_x + {}_1\mathring{q}_x)$. As we are assuming that there are no new entrants or leavers during the 2-year period $_1P_{\{x\}}$ represents the survivors out of $_0P_{\{x-1\}}$ after deducting the corresponding deaths in the first year.

In this idealized problem, therefore, $_0P_{\{x\}}$ and $_1P_{\{x\}}$ are not likely to be very different except at the extreme ages. When new entrants and leavers are allowed for and more than 2 years' experience is combined, the difference between the weighted mean $\mathring{q}_x$ obtained by dividing the total deaths at x by the total exposure at x may be significantly different from the simple average of the separate values of $_t\mathring{q}_x$. In practice, the weighted mean is usually adopted, although for large populations such as the population of England and Wales or the lives assured in the combined experience of the life offices the simple average might just as well be used and, for some purposes, is in fact used. The reasons for adopting the weighted average in practice are: (1) that this process minimizes the resulting random errors, (2) that the combined experience involves much less labour than the process of obtaining the separate values of $_t\mathring{q}_x$ and then averaging them, (3) that separation into years of experience is a quite arbitrary procedure, and (4) that the significant thing for the fund or other organization from which the data have been obtained is usually the total deaths and the combined experience rather than an average mortality rate. If the combined rate is to be used in connexion with a study of the trend in mortality over a long period of years, it must be borne in mind that the average point of time to which the combined experience relates may be significantly different from the mid-point of the period of the experience if $\sum_x {}_tP_x$ is significantly different for different values of t. In any case, in such circumstances the combination of the experience of several years has the effect of reducing the amount of information relevant to the time-trend.

4·3. Exposed-to-risk for several years of experience

Returning now to the expression of $\mathring{q}_x$ for n years of experience combined we note that the numerator represents the deaths at age $\{x\}$ in the n-year period. These can be directly tabulated without segregation into the separate years. We now proceed to show that the exposed-to-risk at each age can be obtained from the census figures at the beginning and end of the period of the investigation together with the numbers of deaths in the period at successive ages, and that the census figures at the beginning of each of the intervening years are not required. It will be seen when we come to consider the adjustments for new entrants and leavers that the same position still obtains provided that the new entrants and leavers during the period are also tabulated in ages. No doubt this convenient result is obvious to some readers, but to many it will be helpful to set out in detail the process by which the intervening census figures cancel out and how the deaths for the individual years of the experience combine into totals for the period for each age.

In considering the exposed-to-risk represented by the combined denominators of the separate values of $_t\hat{q}_x$ we shall assume that the deaths $_t\theta_{\{x\}}$ exactly correspond to the living $_tP_{\{x\}}$. If the correspondence were only approximate, the following procedure would require adjustment in respect of the discrepancy, but as this is ultimately eliminated by the procedure of taking a census at the end of the period of the experience as will emerge later, this complication can be ignored at this stage.

The exposed-to-risk for 1 year is $_0P_{\{x\}}$, and this may be written in the following extended form:

$$E_x = {_0P_{\{x\}}}$$
$$+ {_0P_{\{x-1\}}} - {_1P_{\{x\}}} \quad - {_0\theta_{\{x-1\}}} \quad (\text{i.e.} = 0)$$
$$+ {_0P_{\{x-2\}}} - {_1P_{\{x-1\}}} - {_0\theta_{\{x-2\}}} \quad (\text{i.e.} = 0)$$
$$+ {_0P_{\{x-3\}}} - {_1P_{\{x-2\}}} - {_0\theta_{\{x-3\}}} \quad (\text{i.e.} = 0)$$

down to and including the youngest age.

Therefore
$$E_x = \sum_{x-r}^{x} {_0P_{\{x-r\}}} - \sum_{x-r}^{x} {_1P_{\{x-r\}}} - \sum_{x-r}^{x-1} {_0\theta_{\{x-r\}}}.$$

This expression represents the total population at the beginning of the year up to and including age $\{x\}$ less the total population at the end of the year up to and including age $\{x\}$ less the deaths during the year at all ages up to and including age $\{x-1\}$. A similar extended expression for the second year of a 2-year experience can be written down by substituting the prefixes 1 and 2 for 0 and 1 in the above extended form for the first of the 2 years. We can then add together the expression for the 2 years and reach the following expression for the combined exposed-to-risk at age x for the 2 years:

$$E_x = {}_0P_{\{x\}} + {}_1P_{\{x\}}$$

$$= \sum_{x-r}^{x} {}_0P_{\{x-r\}} - \sum_{x-r}^{x} {}_1P_{\{x-r\}} \qquad - \sum_{x-r}^{x-1} {}_0\theta_{\{x-r\}}$$

$$+ \sum_{x-r}^{x} {}_1P_{\{x-r\}} - \sum_{x-r}^{x} {}_2P_{\{x-r\}} - \sum_{x-r}^{x-1} {}_1\theta_{\{x-r\}}$$

$$= \sum_{x-r}^{x} {}_0P_{\{x-r\}} \qquad - \sum_{x-r}^{x} {}_2P_{\{x-r\}} - \sum_{x-r}^{x-1} \theta_{\{x-r\}}$$

where $\sum_{x-r}^{x-1} \theta_{\{x-r\}}$ is written for $\sum_{x-r}^{x-1} ({}_0\theta_{\{x-r\}} + {}_1\theta_{\{x-r\}})$.

The exposed-to-risk at age x for the 2 years can also be written in a combined extended form as follows, where the items marked A apply to the first year and the items marked B refer to the second year:

$$E_x = {}_0P_{\{x\}} + {}_1P_{\{x\}}$$

$A \quad + {}_0P_{\{x-1\}} - {}_1P_{\{x\}} \qquad - {}_0\theta_{\{x-1\}} \qquad$ (i.e. $=0$)

$B \qquad + {}_1P_{\{x-1\}} - {}_2P_{\{x\}} \qquad - {}_1\theta_{\{x-1\}}$ (i.e. $=0$)

$A \quad + {}_0P_{\{x-2\}} - {}_1P_{\{x-1\}} \qquad - {}_0\theta_{\{x-2\}} \qquad$ (i.e. $=0$)

$B \qquad + {}_1P_{\{x-2\}} - {}_2P_{\{x-1\}} \qquad - {}_1\theta_{\{x-2\}}$ (i.e. $=0$)

$A \quad + {}_0P_{\{x-3\}} - {}_1P_{\{x-2\}} \qquad - {}_0\theta_{\{x-3\}} \qquad$ (i.e. $=0$)

$$\vdots \qquad \vdots \qquad \vdots \qquad \vdots$$

down to and including the youngest age.

Therefore

$$E_x = \sum_{x-r}^{x} {}_0P_{\{x-r\}} - \sum_{x-r}^{x} {}_2P_{\{x-r\}} - \sum_{x-r}^{x-1} {}_0\theta_{\{x-r\}} - \sum_{x-r}^{x-1} {}_1\theta_{\{x-r\}}$$

$$= \sum_{x-r}^{x} {}_0P_{\{x-r\}} - \sum_{x-r}^{x} {}_2P_{\{x-r\}} - \sum_{x-r}^{x-1} \theta_{\{x-r\}}.$$

This expression represents the total population at the beginning of the 2-year period up to and including age $\{x\}$ less the total population at the end of the 2-year period up to and including age $\{x\}$ less the deaths during the 2-year period at all ages up to and including age $\{x-1\}$. It should be noted that the symbol $\theta_{\{x\}}$ without a prefix is used for all the deaths in the period of the experience at age x, viz. $\theta_{\{x-1\}} = {}_0\theta_{\{x-1\}} + {}_1\theta_{\{x-1\}}$ for a 2-year period.

Evidently the same system applies for a 3-year period and generally for an n-year period, but it may be helpful to write out in extended form the exposed-to-risk for a 3-year period, marking the items A, B and C respectively for the first, second and third years. The exposed-to-risk at age x for 3 years is thus:

$$E_x = {}_0P_{\{x\}} + {}_1P_{\{x\}} + {}_2P_{\{x\}}$$
$$A \quad + {}_0P_{\{x-1\}} - {}_1P_{\{x\}} \qquad\qquad - {}_0\theta_{\{x-1\}}$$
$$B \qquad\qquad + {}_1P_{\{x-1\}} - {}_2P_{\{x\}} \qquad\qquad - {}_1\theta_{\{x-1\}}$$
$$C \qquad\qquad\qquad + {}_2P_{\{x-1\}} - {}_3P_{\{x\}} \qquad\qquad - {}_2\theta_{\{x-1\}}$$
$$A \quad + {}_0P_{\{x-2\}} - {}_1P_{\{x-1\}} \qquad\qquad - {}_0\theta_{\{x-2\}}$$
$$B \qquad\qquad + {}_1P_{\{x-2\}} - {}_2P_{\{x-1\}} \qquad\qquad - {}_1\theta_{\{x-2\}}$$
$$C \qquad\qquad\qquad + {}_2P_{\{x-2\}} - {}_3P_{\{x-1\}} \qquad\qquad - {}_2\theta_{\{x-2\}}$$
$$\vdots \qquad \vdots \qquad \vdots \qquad \vdots \qquad \vdots \qquad \vdots \qquad \vdots$$

down to and including the youngest age.

Therefore
$$E_x = \sum_{x-r}^{x} {}_0P_{\{x-r\}} - \sum_{x-r}^{x} {}_3P_{\{x-r\}} - \sum_{x-r}^{x-1} \theta_{\{x-r\}}.$$

It will be observed how in the above scheme all the population enumerations between the beginning and the end of the period of the experience cancel out, and how the deaths for the separate years combine into total deaths for each age and for all ages up to age $\{x-1\}$. Indeed, it was solely in order to exhibit this process of cancellation of the intermediate enumerations and this combination of the deaths that the extended form of expression of the exposed-to-risk was set out in detail.

For an investigation over n years the exposed-to-risk at age x thus takes the form

$$\sum_{x-r}^{x} {}_0P_{\{x-r\}} - \sum_{x-r}^{x} {}_nP_{\{x-r\}} - \sum_{x-r}^{x-1} \theta_{\{x-r\}}.$$

A proper appreciation of the reason for the identity of the two forms of the exposed-to-risk at age x for an n-year experience

$$\left(\text{i.e. } \sum_{t=0}^{n-1} {}_t P_{\{x\}} = \sum_{x-r}^{x} {}_0 P_{\{x-r\}} - \sum_{x-r}^{x} {}_n P_{\{x-r\}} - \sum_{x-r}^{x-1} \theta_{\{x-r\}}\right)$$

is fundamental to a proper understanding of the technique of exposed-to-risk formulae. At the risk of repetition and of labouring the discussion, but to help those students who, experience has shown, do not find the identity immediately obvious, we proceed to explain what to some readers is, no doubt, already obvious. Still assuming that there are no new entrants or leavers, the exposed-to-risk $\sum_{t=0}^{n-1} {}_t P_{\{x\}}$ represents all those who enter on the year of age $\{x\}$ to $\{x+1\}$ during the n-year period (e.g. all those who (1) reach their xth birthdays during the period if life years are being used or (2) are aged x nearest on 1 January of one of the years of the n-year period if calendar years and nearest ages are being used). Similarly, all those who are aged $\{x\}$ or under at the commencement of the period (i.e. $\sum_{x-r}^{x} {}_0 P_{\{x-r\}}$) must reach age $\{x\}$ during the period unless they die at age $\{x-1\}$ or earlier, i.e. $\sum_{x-r}^{x-1} \theta_{\{x-r\}}$, or survive the period but are so young that they have not by then passed age $\{x\}$, i.e. $\sum_{x-r}^{x} {}_n P_{\{x-r\}}$. The exposed-to-risk at x is thus all those who enter the experience at $\{x\}$ or under less all those who die before $\{x\}$ or leave the experience at or before reaching $\{x\}$.

If the living and deaths are tabulated in a form such that there is only an approximate correspondence between them, the principles of the identity of the two forms of the exposed-to-risk still apply. The only difference is that in the extended form of the exposed-to-risk the deaths in each identity of the form ${}_t P_{x-r} - {}_{t+1} P_{x-r+1} - {}_t \theta_{x-r} = 0$ must be those which strictly correspond to the living at the beginning and end of the year *and not the deaths as tabulated*. The deaths as tabulated are used for the numerators of the mortality rates; the yearly census figures ${}_t P_{\{x-r\}}$ in one form of the exposed-to-risk and the terminal census figures ${}_0 P_{\{x-r\}}$ and ${}_n P_{\{x-r\}}$ in the other form do not depend on the tabulated deaths. The deductive item $\sum_{x-r}^{x-1} \theta_{\{x-r\}}$ in the second form, in principle, refers to the deaths that strictly correspond to the living. In practice, however, this item will usually be based on the tabulated deaths, and so there will be a small discrepancy. This discrepancy will usually be confined to the last term contained in $\sum_{x-r}^{x-1} \theta_{\{x-r\}}$ which refers to the deaths at age $\{x-1\}$, since the discrepancies between the strictly corresponding deaths and the tabulated deaths at the earlier ages will have cancelled themselves out by discrepancies of opposite signs at adjacent ages, that is to say, all the deaths at ages $x-2$ and earlier, however tabulated, will be included at one or other of the ages up to and including $\{x-1\}$ in the other tabulation. For example, if the living are tabulated according to nearest ages on 1 January and the deaths are tabulated at ages last birthday at death, the deductive item $\sum_{x-r}^{x-1} \theta_{x-r}$ based on the tabulated deaths will include all the deaths out of the exposed-to-risk at all nearest ages up to $\{x-2\}$, since the maximum age last birthday at death for these deaths is $x-1$.

4·4. Notation for continuous exposed-to-risk formulae

We now introduce the more usual notation for exposed-to-risk formulae:

$E_x =$ the exposed-to-risk at age x,

$b_x =$ the number living at the beginning of the period of the investigation at assumed integral age x (b stands for beginners),

$e_x =$ the number living at the end of the period of the investigation at assumed integral age x (e stands for existing or enders).

b_x and e_x correspond to $_0P_{\{x\}}$ and $_nP_{\{x\}}$ in the previous notation, and in both symbols the x is some approximation, on the average, to the integral age, e.g. nearest age or age next birthday at entry plus curtate duration. There is now no need to put brackets round the x as for the population symbol where it was necessary to distinguish

P_x ($=$ population at age x last birthday) and

$P_{\{x\}}$ ($=$ population at assumed exact age x, on the average),

$\theta_x =$ the total number of deaths during the period of the investigation at age x last birthday (or at assumed age x last birthday, e.g. nearest age at the beginning of the year of death).

The brackets may be used for $\theta_{\{x\}}$ to indicate when the age is not the actual age last birthday at death but an assumed age at the beginning of the year of death, when this is a calendar year or a policy year.

In this notation the exposed-to-risk at age x, i.e. from exact age x to exact age $x+1$, is

$$E_x = \sum_{x-r}^{x} b_{x-r} - \sum_{x-r}^{x} e_{x-r} - \sum_{x-r}^{x-1} \theta_{\{x-r\}}.$$

Since
$$E_{x-1} = \sum_{x-r}^{x-1} b_{x-r} - \sum_{x-r}^{x-1} e_{x-r} - \sum_{x-r}^{x-2} \theta_{\{x-r\}},$$

$$E_x = E_{x-1} + b_x - e_x - \theta_{\{x-1\}}.$$

This exposed-to-risk is for the q-type of mortality rate so that

$$\mathring{q}_x \doteqdot \theta_{\{x\}}/E_x.$$

For the m-type of mortality rate we require the exposed-to-risk in central form and this is readily obtained from E_x by deducting one-half of the deaths that form the numerator of $\mathring{q}_x$ so that

$$E_x^c = E_x - \tfrac{1}{2}\theta_{\{x\}}$$
$$= E_{x-1}^c + b_x - e_x - \tfrac{1}{2}(\theta_{\{x-1\}} + \theta_{\{x\}})$$

and
$$\mathring{m}_x \doteqdot \theta_{\{x\}}/E_x^c.$$

These exposed-to-risk formulae are called 'continuous' formulae because they enable the exposed-to-risk at successive ages to be computed by a continuous process, starting at the youngest age α, obtaining $E_{\alpha+1}$ from E_α, $E_{\alpha+2}$ from $E_{\alpha+1}$ and so on. The word 'continuous' is not very apt, and it would be preferable to call the formulae 'difference' formulae since they are really expressions for ΔE_{x-1}. In the Σ-form E_x is seen to be equal to the sum of all 'beginners' at ages up to and including age x less the sum of all 'enders' at ages up to and including age x less the sum of all deaths at ages last birthday up to and including age $x-1$. The significance of the treatment of the deaths should be especially noticed. As in a 1-year experience all the deaths in the year of death are included as a full unit in the exposed-to-risk, that is, they are given *a full year's exposure in the year of death*.

For the central rate, on the other hand, the deaths should be exposed only up to the exact age at death, since

$$m_x = \frac{d_x}{L_x} = d_x \bigg/ \int_0^1 l_{x+t} dt.$$

For E_x^c the deaths are therefore given only a half-year's exposure in the year of death which, on the assumption of a uniform distribution of the deaths over the year, is equivalent, on the average, to exposing them only up to the actual age at death.

4·5. The total exposure and the allocation over the ages

It will be observed that if, in an *n*-year investigation, a life is included in b_x and in e_{x+n} the continuous exposed-to-risk formulae automatically ensure that it appears in each of E_x, E_{x+1}, ..., E_{x+n-1}, that is, it is exposed in exactly *n* ages and therefore given exactly *n* years of exposure. This is, of course, exactly what is required in total. The only possible point of doubt is whether the exposure appears at the right ages. If the assumed ages at the beginning and end of the period of the investigation are reasonably accurate the only doubt about the ages to which the exposure is allocated is at the first and last ages, i.e. at x and $x+n-1$. The life is correctly exposed at ages $x+1$ to $x+n-2$, both inclusive. If x is the nearest age a particular life may be, in actual fact, exposed for only a part of the year of age x to $x+1$. By giving such cases a full year's exposure at age x they are being averaged with other cases which, because they are treated as x exact or $x+1$ exact when their exact ages are, in fact, $x-k$ and $x+1-k$, are given insufficient exposure at ages $x-1$ and x respectively. Similar considerations apply to the ages $x+n$ at the end of the period. The accuracy of any exposed-to-risk formula thus turns on the suitability of the averaging assumptions made for the ages of the beginners and enders. As will be seen in the next chapter similar considerations also apply to the approximations used for the ages of the new entrants and the leavers. If a life is included in b_x and in θ_{x+s-1} the continuous exposed-to-risk formulae automatically include it in each of E_x, E_{x+1}, ..., E_{x+s-1}, i.e. the life is exposed at s ages for s full years.

The beginners, enders, deaths (and new entrants and leavers) can be tabulated in ages defined in a variety of ways and in a variety of mixtures of ways, e.g. b_x may be tabulated according to nearest ages and new entrants according to ages next birthday. Each problem of this kind requires a suitable continuous exposed-to-risk formula to be devised with proper regard to the form in which the ages are defined. Details of such formulae are outside the scope of this book; the subject will be taken up in more detail and more generally, particularly in relation to selection and multiple-decrement problems, in Volume II.

For the present, it should be emphasized that for any exposed-to-risk formula to be satisfactory it must achieve two separate and distinct ends which should always be kept sharply in mind. It must ensure that the total exposed-to-risk is accurate; and it must allocate this total appropriately over the individual ages.

4·6. An example, with a checking system

The continuous process of building up E_x from E_{x-1} by summation from the top of a table of beginners, enders and deaths ensures that at the oldest age $E_x = 0$. This is illustrated in the example given in Table 4·1. As a rough check on the whole process the following approximate relation should apply

$$\Sigma E_x \doteqdot \tfrac{1}{2} n (\Sigma b_x + \Sigma e_x) + \tfrac{1}{2} \Sigma \theta_x,$$

where n is the number of years in the experience. By taking the mean between Σb_x and Σe_x and multiplying by n we give all those persisting throughout the whole period exactly n years' exposure and all the deaths $\tfrac{1}{2} n$ years' exposure. As this takes the deaths, on the average, only up to the date of death we must give them all another half-year's exposure. The discrepancy between the two sides of the above approximate relation should be confined solely to the effect which comes from the deaths not being uniformly spread over the n years. A complete check can, therefore, be made by tabulating

TABLE 4·1. *Example of the continuous exposed-to-risk formula* $E_x = E_{x-1} + b_x - e_x - \theta_{\{x-1\}}$ *applied to a 5-year experience.*

x	E_x	b_x	e_x	$\theta_{\{x\}}$
60	179	179	—	3
1	368	192	—	7
2	522	161	—	14
3	650	142	—	15
4	767	132	—	16
65	722	134	163	18
6	658	126	172	21
7	610	116	143	19
8	572	104	123	23
9	529	92	112	17
70	475	74	111	20
1	407	62	110	17
2	342	41	89	22
3	260	23	83	19
4	179	16	78	14
75	124	8	49	9
6	70	—	45	6
7	37	—	27	1
8	21	—	15	3
9	6	—	12	1
80	—	—	5	—
Total	7498	1602	1337	265

the deaths at all ages for each year of the experience separately, and this procedure is well worth doing. It will be seen later that a similar procedure is possible when allowance is made for new entrants and leavers.

4·7. Summing from the other end

In a mortality table l_x can be regarded as the 'expected' survivors at age x out of l_α entrants at age α. Before age α, $l_x = 0$; after ω, l_x again $= 0$. l_x can be obtained by continuous summation from the top or from the bottom of the deaths column, i.e.

$$l_x = l_\alpha - \sum_{x-r}^{x-1} {}_\alpha d_{x-r}$$

$$= \sum_{x+r}^{\omega} {}_x d_{x+r}.$$

Similarly, since E_x is obtained by continuous summation and since it starts at o at the youngest age and finishes at o at the oldest age, the whole process could be carried out by summing continuously from the bottom of the column of beginners, enders and deaths instead of from the top. The reason for this can be seen from the fact that the exposed-to-risk at age x must be equal to all those who die at age x, plus all those who leave or die at age $x + 1$ or over, less all those who begin at age $x + 1$ or over. In symbols we have

$$E_x = \sum_r {}_1 e_{x+r} - \sum_r {}_1 b_{x+r} + \sum_r {}_0 \theta_{x+r}.$$

In fact, a table in the form of the example in §4·6 can be treated as if it were a multiple 'increment and decrement' table with E_x as equivalent to l_x. The arithmetical analogy would be complete if the ages for b_x and e_x were last birthday as for θ_x. It would not, of course, be right to pursue the analogy into the field of interpretation because the meaning and purposes of the two tables are significantly different. Let us define l_x as the number of lives reaching exact age x while in the group at any time during the period of observation, and b_x, e_x and θ_x as the numbers of beginners, enders and deaths during the period of observation, all at age x last birthday. Then, since those reaching age x must be equal to those reaching age $x - 1$ plus those entering between $x - 1$ and x less those leaving or dying between $x - 1$ and x, we have

$$l_x = l_{x-1} + b_{x-1} - e_{x-1} - \theta_{x-1}.$$

The enumerations l_x may be regarded as a kind of 'dynamic census' in contrast to the enumerations ${}_tP_x$ at the particular point of time t, and further reference to this notion appears in §§5·8 and 5·10. Now if we assume that b_x and e_x are uniformly spread over the year of age we should expose them for half a year in the year of age x to $x + 1$. Hence
$$E_x = l_x + \tfrac{1}{2} b_x - \tfrac{1}{2} e_x$$
and
$$\mathring{q}_x \doteqdot \theta_x / (l_x + \tfrac{1}{2} b_x - \tfrac{1}{2} e_x),$$
$$\mathring{m}_x \doteqdot \theta_x / (l_x + \tfrac{1}{2} b_x - \tfrac{1}{2} e_x - \tfrac{1}{2} \theta_x).$$

Alternatively, by averaging the deaths between successive ages an approximation to the central rates at half-ages is given by

$$\mathring{m}_{x-\frac{1}{2}} \doteqdot \tfrac{1}{2} (\theta_{x-1} + \theta_x) / l_x.$$

This arithmetical analogy will be extended to include new entrants and leavers in the next chapter and will be pursued further in Volume II, first in developing, in more detail, continuous exposed-to-risk formulae when the ages are given in various different ways and then in relation to the subject of multiple-decrement tables.

4·8. The census method

It has been shown earlier how the census method for a 1-year experience can be expressed in the same form as an ordinary exposed-to-risk formula. This could also be done for a combined experience for several years. But in practical life-office work the census method is usually applied for each year separately and combined results are then obtained by direct combination. This is because the census totals for each age (and for each duration separately up to, say, 5 years) are tabulated as at the end of each calendar year. These totals are built up continuously as part of the machinery of the classification of the policies for valuation purposes. This process will be described more fully after discussing the adjustments for new entrants and leavers. For the present it is sufficient to indicate the process of combination. Thus if

$$_t\mathring{q}_x \doteqdot {}_t\theta_x / \tfrac{1}{2}({}_tP_x + {}_{t+1}P_x + {}_t\theta_x)$$

and

$$_t\mathring{m}_x \doteqdot {}_t\theta_x / \tfrac{1}{2}({}_tP_x + {}_{t+1}P_x),$$

the combined rate of mortality for n years is

$$\mathring{q}_x \doteqdot \sum_{t=0}^{n-1} {}_t\theta_x \left/ \frac{1}{2}\left(\sum_{t=0}^{n-1} {}_tP_x + \sum_{t=1}^{n} {}_tP_x + \sum_{t=0}^{n-1} {}_t\theta_x\right)\right.$$

$$\doteqdot \sum_{t=0}^{n-1} {}_t\theta_x \left/ \left(\tfrac{1}{2}\,{}_0P_x + \sum_{t=1}^{n-1} {}_tP_x + \tfrac{1}{2}\,{}_nP_x + \tfrac{1}{2}\sum_{t=0}^{n-1} {}_t\theta_x\right)\right.,$$

$$\mathring{m}_x \doteqdot \sum_{t=0}^{n-1} {}_t\theta_x \left/ \left(\tfrac{1}{2}\,{}_0P_x + \sum_{t=1}^{n-1} {}_tP_x + \tfrac{1}{2}\,{}_nP_x\right)\right..$$

CHAPTER 5

ADJUSTMENTS FOR NEW ENTRANTS AND LEAVERS

5·1. Selection excluded from consideration

In discussing the various procedures for obtaining rates of mortality, both for a group as a whole and for individual ages or durations, it has so far been assumed that, during the period of the investigation, the group has been a closed group subject only to depletion by death. This is, of course, an unrealistic situation, but it has been assumed in order to simplify the discussion of the basic principles of mortality investigations. The effect of lives joining and leaving the group during the period of the investigation and the adjustments necessary to allow for them do not raise any important questions of principle as long as it is assumed that neither the new entrants nor the leavers form a 'select' class of lives, i.e. as long as it is assumed that their mortality rates, apart from random errors, do not differ from the mortality rates of the group or subgroup which they join or leave. The implications of 'heterogeneity' and 'selection' are, however, excluded from discussion in this book; they will be taken up in Volume II. The only questions arising for consideration at this stage, therefore, are the adjustments to be made in the exposed-to-risk formulae to allow for new entrants and leavers on the assumption of homogeneity as between the new entrants, leavers and the relevant subgroup.

5·2. New entrants

In an investigation extending over a single calendar year or over the period from the birthday in one calendar year to the birthday in the next calendar year, there are two courses open to us for dealing with new entrants during the year of observation. We could ignore the new entrants entirely, in which event any deaths that occur during the year among the new entrants must also be rigorously excluded from the number of deaths. The process of obtaining rates of mortality is then the same as if there were no new entrants.

Alternatively, an approximate allowance could be made for the fractions of the year during which the new entrants are included in the group and hence are exposed to the risk of death; the deaths among the new entrants would then also be included in the number of deaths. The basis of the approximate allowance usually made is the assumption that, for a given number of lives all exposed for the full year, the corresponding deaths would, apart from random fluctuations, be uniformly spread over the year. In practice, this is usually a good enough assumption for the purpose, although when rates analysed by age are required the assumption is known to be untrue. From the general shape of the function $(\mu l)_x$ of many mortality tables based on actual mortality data we know that for adult ages up to the middle seventies the expected number of deaths in the second half of a year of age is greater than the expected number for the first half of the year. The reverse position applies at the older ages after the middle seventies and at the infantile ages, and sometimes $(\mu l)_x$ falls slightly over a short age-range in the twenties. Nevertheless, if, for example, four lives enter the experience at age $x + \frac{3}{4}$ it is usually accurate enough to treat them as one life exposed throughout the year of age x to $x + 1$. In fact, a more approximate treatment still is usually accorded to the new entrants by assuming that their entry dates are uniformly spread over the observation year. Thus by giving half of the new entrants a full year's exposure or, what is the same thing on the assumptions made, by giving them all half a year's exposure, we can approximate to the total of the actual fractional periods of exposure.

If $_0P_{\{x\}}$ is the number starting the year (whether a life year or a calendar year) at assumed integral age x, and $n_{\{x\}}$ is the number of new entrants whose assumed integral age at the beginning of the observation year was x, and $\theta_{\{x\}}$ is the number of the corresponding deaths (including those among the new entrants), then the adjusted formulae for the rates of mortality, assuming that there are no leavers, would be as follows:

$$\mathring{q}_x \doteqdot \theta_{\{x\}}/(_0P_{\{x\}} + \tfrac{1}{2}n_{\{x\}}),$$

$$\mathring{m}_x \doteqdot \theta_{\{x\}}/(_0P_{\{x\}} + \tfrac{1}{2}n_{\{x\}} - \tfrac{1}{2}\theta_{\{x\}}).$$

There are various other ways of treating the new entrants. For example, we might give a full year's exposure to the entrants in the first half of the year of observation and no exposure at all to the entrants in the second half of the year. Another way would be for the ages of the new entrants to be based on the actual ages at the time of entry. If the ages for $_0P_{(x)}$ were nearest ages and the ages for θ were ages last birthday at death (so that the deaths and the living would not exactly correspond), the new entrants might be tabulated at their nearest integral ages at the date of entry. Since they would be assumed to enter, on the average, in the middle of the observation year they would each be exposed for half a year at the ages assigned to them. The formulae for the mortality rates would still be as shown above subject to the appropriate meanings being attached to $\{x\}$ in the respective symbols. If this course were followed, however, some of the deaths out of the entrants at nearest age x would be included as deaths at age $x-1$, and some of the deaths out of the entrants at nearest age $x+1$ would be included as deaths at age x. Although this would add to the degree of non-correspondence between the living and the deaths there would usually be a reasonably adequate balancing effect between the successive ages.

To achieve a closer, but still not a complete correspondence for the new entrants, it might be worth while to assign $\frac{1}{4}n_x$ to age $x-1$ and $\frac{3}{4}n_x$ to age x. The basis of these complementary fractions is the assumption that $\frac{1}{2}n_x$ enter, on the average, at age $x-\frac{1}{4}$ (since $x=$ nearest age at entry), so that half of their assumed half-year of exposure is in the year of age $x-1$ and the other half in the year of age x; the other half of n_x would then be assumed to enter, on the average, at age $x+\frac{1}{4}$, so that the whole of their assumed half-year of exposure would be in the year of age x. On this basis the formula for the rate of mortality for one observation year would be

$$\mathring{q}_x = \theta_x / (_0P_{\{x\}} + \tfrac{3}{8}n_x + \tfrac{1}{8}n_{x+1}).$$

This kind of meticulous respreading of the ages of the new entrants to achieve a closer correspondence with the deaths is, however, usually not worth doing. Strictly, an adjustment should also be made to allow for the fact that the ratio of the deaths among the new entrants to one-half of the new entrants gives an approximation to $2 \times {}_{\frac{1}{2}}q_x$ rather than to q_x. The assumption that

$$(l_x - l_{x+\frac{1}{2}})/l_x \quad \text{is equal to} \quad \tfrac{1}{2}(l_x - l_{x+1})/l_x$$

is, however, equivalent to assuming a uniform spread of the deaths over the year of age, and for practical purposes it is usually an adequate approximation, particularly when considered with the other assumptions made, e.g. that the new entrants, on the average, enter at the middle of the observation year.

Whatever process is used for allocating the new entrants and the deaths over the respective ages, the overriding necessity is to ensure that, for the entire set of rates, the total of the exposed-to-risk, summed over all the ages, allows the right amount of exposure to new entrants. If it is being assumed that the new entrants are, on the average, exposed for half a year, the total exposed-to-risk for the set of $\hat{q}$'s for one observation year must equal $\Sigma_0 P_{(x)} + \frac{1}{2}\Sigma n_x$, and for the corresponding set of $\hat{m}$'s the total must equal

$$\Sigma_0 P_{(x)} + \tfrac{1}{2}\Sigma n_x - \tfrac{1}{2}\Sigma \theta_x.$$

5·3. Policy years

If the investigation is being made from the policy anniversary in one calendar year to the policy anniversary in the next, the new entrants in the first calendar year would clearly be exposed for a full year, while the new entrants in the second calendar year would not be exposed at all. The treatment of the deaths would correspond in the observation year. If mortality rates for separate years of duration were being extracted, the new entrants in the first calendar year would comprise $E_{[x]}$, where x might be the nearest age at entry or the calendar-year age at entry (i.e. calendar year of entry less calendar year of birth). Alternatively, the entry age might be age next birthday, in which case the ratio to $E_{[x]}$ of the deaths out of the corresponding new entrants at age x next birthday would provide an approximation to $\hat{q}_{[x-\frac{1}{2}]}$ on the assumption that the entries are uniformly spread between birthdays.

For lives assured the average age of those entering at age x next birthday might well be greater than $x - \frac{1}{2}$ owing to the tendency to effect policies just before a birthday, although this is offset to some extent by a tendency for more policies to be effected just before the end of a calendar year than just after. This feature, in its turn, however, has a correspondingly disturbing effect on the validity of such approximations as the calendar-year age for the average age at entry or the curtate duration plus half a year for the average duration on 1 January. These difficulties are rarely of sufficient importance to call for special treatment, but their existence should always be kept in mind when making assumptions about average ages, average durations and average periods of exposure.

For annuitants there used to be a strong tendency for the annuities to be bought just after a birthday and, in fact, investigation showed that the average age of those recorded as entering at age x last birthday was approximately $x + \frac{1}{3}$. Nowadays, however, many offices quote annuity purchase prices for each half-age and some quote for quarter-ages, so that the disturbing effect of these discrete changes in the purchase-price tables has become much reduced.

5·4. Leavers

An adjustment of the exposed-to-risk similar to that for new entrants is necessary for those leaving the experience during the year of observation otherwise than by death, but in this case the adjustment takes the form of excluding part of a year's exposure for each leaver in respect of the period after the date of leaving. As has been mentioned, it is possible to evade the problem for the new entrants by entirely excluding them and the corresponding deaths, but we cannot do this for the leavers because we cannot say which of the deaths would have been leavers if they had not died!

Those leaving the experience may do so for various reasons, according to the nature of the group whose mortality is being examined. For a general population experience the leavers would comprise the emigrants; the immigrants would, of course, be new entrants. This would apply also to the local migrants for sectional experiences. In an occupational experience those entering or leaving a particular occupation would be the new entrants and leavers for that occupation. In all these cases it is usually appropriate to assume that the migrations are uniformly spread over the year of observation so that, to obtain the exposed-to-risk, the number living at the beginning of the year must be increased by half the immigrants and diminished by half the emigrants. Using the symbol w (= withdrawals) for the emigrants and assuming that the ages are all based on age last birthday on 1 January of the calendar year of observation, the rates of mortality could be obtained by the formulae

$$\mathring{q}_{x-\frac{1}{2}} \doteqdot \theta_{(x-\frac{1}{2})}/({}_0P_{x-1} + \tfrac{1}{2}n_{(x-\frac{1}{2})} - \tfrac{1}{2}w_{(x-\frac{1}{2})}),$$

$$\mathring{m}_{x-\frac{1}{2}} \doteqdot \theta_{(x-\frac{1}{2})}/({}_0P_{x-1} + \tfrac{1}{2}n_{(x-\frac{1}{2})} - \tfrac{1}{2}w_{(x-\frac{1}{2})} - \tfrac{1}{2}\theta_{(x-\frac{1}{2})}).$$

Now the population at age x last birthday at the end of the year is equal to the population at age $x - 1$ last birthday at the beginning of the year plus the corresponding new entrants and less the corresponding leavers and deaths, viz.

$$_1P_x = {}_0P_{x-1} + n_{(x-\frac{1}{2})} - w_{(x-\frac{1}{2})} - \theta_{(x-\frac{1}{2})},$$

so that

$$\mathring{q}_{x-\frac{1}{2}} \doteqdot \theta_{(x-\frac{1}{2})}/\tfrac{1}{2}({}_0P_{x-1} + {}_1P_x + \theta_{(x-\frac{1}{2})}),$$

$$\mathring{m}_{x-\frac{1}{2}} \doteqdot \theta_{(x-\frac{1}{2})}/\tfrac{1}{2}({}_0P_{x-1} + {}_1P_x).$$

Since the deaths $\theta_{(x-\frac{1}{2})}$ were all aged $x - 1$ last birthday on 1 January, their ages at death range from $x - 1$ to $x + 1$ and are centred on x. Similarly, the ages at death for $\theta_{(x+\frac{1}{2})}$ are centred on $x + 1$ and so on. It would, therefore, be a reasonable approximation to substitute the deaths at nearest age x at death for $\theta_{(x-\frac{1}{2})}$ in both the numerator and the denominator of $\mathring{q}_{x-\frac{1}{2}}$ and in the numerator of $\mathring{m}_{x-\frac{1}{2}}$.

The expression $\tfrac{1}{2}({}_0P_{x-1} + {}_1P_x)$ in the denominators of the rates is, clearly, an approximation to the population at nearest age x on 1 July, since we are assuming that all the changes are uniformly spread over the year. Given a census on 1 July, therefore, the rates of mortality may be obtained from

$$\mathring{q}_{x-\frac{1}{2}} \doteqdot \theta_{x-\frac{1}{2}}/(\tfrac{1}{2}P_{x-\frac{1}{2}} + \tfrac{1}{2}\theta_{x-\frac{1}{2}}),$$

$$\mathring{m}_{x-\frac{1}{2}} \doteqdot \theta_{x-\frac{1}{2}}/\tfrac{1}{2}P_{x-\frac{1}{2}},$$

where $\theta_{x-\frac{1}{2}}$ is the number of deaths at the nearest age x at death and $\tfrac{1}{2}P_{x-\frac{1}{2}}$ is the number living at nearest age x on 1 July. Similarly, if the census ages and the ages at death were x last birthday the mortality rates would be given by

$$\mathring{q}_x \doteqdot \theta_x/(\tfrac{1}{2}P_x + \tfrac{1}{2}\theta_x),$$

$$\mathring{m}_x \doteqdot \theta_x/\tfrac{1}{2}P_x.$$

If the year of observation is a policy year the corresponding procedure would be to enumerate the living on 1 January between the policy anniversaries either (a) at ages last birthday or (b), if select rates are required, according to curtate duration and assumed entry ages (e.g. nearest integral age at entry). The mortality rates for (a) would then be

$$\mathring{q}_x \doteqdot \theta_x/(P_x + \tfrac{1}{2}\theta_x),$$

$$\mathring{m}_x \doteqdot \theta_x/P_x,$$

where $x =$ age last birthday and P_x is the enumeration on 1 January.

The mortality rates for (b) would be

$$\mathring{q}_{[x]+t} \doteqdot \theta_{[x]+t}/(P_{[x]+t} + \tfrac{1}{2}\theta_{[x]+t})$$

$$\doteqdot \theta_{[x]+t}/(P_{[x]+t} + \theta^\alpha_{[x]+t}),$$

$$\mathring{m}_{[x]+t} \doteqdot \theta_{[x]+t}/P_{[x]+t},$$

where $x =$ nearest age at entry, $t =$ curtate duration and $P_{[x]+t}$ is the enumeration on 1 January; $\theta^\alpha_{[x]+t}$ represents the deaths before 1 January that are included in $\theta_{[x]+t}$.

It will be observed that this procedure averages the exposure for the leavers between policy anniversaries. It also uses census data in select form to provide rates of mortality for integral durations with a complete correspondence between the deaths and the living. This procedure was first suggested by A. T. Haynes (*J.I.A.* **69**, 153), but it has never been adopted for the British Offices' continuous investigations.

5·5. The census method

An approximation to the number of living at age x last birthday on 1 July can be obtained by taking the mean between the numbers living at age x last birthday at the beginning and at the end of the calendar year, viz.

$$\tfrac{1}{2}P_x \doteqdot \tfrac{1}{2}({}_0P_x + {}_1P_x),$$

and this expression may also be interpreted as the mean population at age x last birthday throughout the year. Thus we arrive at the typical 'census-method' formulae

$$\mathring{q}_x \doteqdot \theta_x / \tfrac{1}{2}({}_0P_x + {}_1P_x + \theta_x),$$
$$\mathring{m}_x \doteqdot \theta_x / \tfrac{1}{2}({}_0P_x + {}_1P_x),$$

where $x = $ age last birthday, and

$$\mathring{q}_{x-\frac{1}{2}} \doteqdot \theta_{x-\frac{1}{2}} / \tfrac{1}{2}({}_0P_{x-\frac{1}{2}} + {}_1P_{x-\frac{1}{2}} + \theta_{x-\frac{1}{2}}),$$
$$\mathring{m}_{x-\frac{1}{2}} \doteqdot \theta_{x-\frac{1}{2}} / \tfrac{1}{2}({}_0P_{x-\frac{1}{2}} + {}_1P_{x-\frac{1}{2}}),$$

where $x - \tfrac{1}{2}$ is age 'last birthday' which is, of course, equivalent to age x nearest birthday.

For select rates the enumerations on 1 January would be in respect of curtate durations. The deaths would also be recorded for curtate durations. The ages might be ages last birthday both for the censuses and for the deaths, or they might be nearest ages for both. Taking the latter as an illustration, the following rates of mortality result:

$$\mathring{q}_{[x-t-\frac{1}{2}]+t} \doteqdot \theta_{x,t} / \tfrac{1}{2}({}_0P_{x,t} + {}_1P_{x,t} + \theta_{x,t}),$$
$$\mathring{m}_{[x-t-\frac{1}{2}]+t} \doteqdot \theta_{x,t} / \tfrac{1}{2}({}_0P_{x,t} + {}_1P_{x,t}).$$

These are the formulae used in the British Offices' continuous investigations of assured lives and annuitants.

All these census formulae allow half a year's exposure for each new entrant and for each leaver. It should be noted that for these 'census-method' formulae there is not necessarily a strict correspondence between the deaths and the exposed-to-risk. It will also be noted that in all these formulae the total of the numerators over all ages is $\Sigma\theta$, the total of the denominators for q is

$$\tfrac{1}{2}(\Sigma_0 P + \Sigma_1 P + \Sigma\theta) \quad \text{or} \quad (\Sigma_{\frac{1}{2}}P + \tfrac{1}{2}\Sigma\theta),$$

and the total of the denominators for m is

$$\tfrac{1}{2}(\Sigma_0 P + \Sigma_1 P) \quad \text{or} \quad (\Sigma_{\frac{1}{2}}P).$$

5·6. Various kinds of leavers

In an experience of annuitants there are usually no leavers because offices do not usually allow annuities to be surrendered for cash. For other groups of lives, however, there may be various different kinds of leavers. They are not all withdrawals in the usual sense of the word 'withdrawal', and that is why the general word 'leaver' has been used instead of the more commonly used word 'withdrawal'.

In a pension fund the leavers include those members who withdraw from the fund because they have left the employ of the organization for which the fund is maintained. There will also be those who retire on pension because of ill-health, those who retire on 'optional pension' before the normal retirement age, and those who retire on pension at the normal retirement age. For a mortality experience of the members 'in service' all these are leavers, but the different categories may require separate treatment, quite apart from the fact that they may play the part of new entrants into separate mortality experiences of ill-health pensioners and of normal pensioners. If there is any concentration of retirement at particular points of age (e.g. on attaining age 60 or age 65) or at particular points of time (e.g. at the end of calendar years), the usual assumptions regarding uniformity of spread over years of age or over calendar years would be inappropriate and other suitable approximations would need to be devised. In practice, the experience of a pension fund is often directed to producing a multiple-decrement table, and the special considerations then arising are outside the scope of the present volume. To complete the general picture it may be mentioned that an experience of a pension fund might conceivably be segregated into different grades of staff so that promotion, and demotion, would represent leavers from one grade and new entrants to another. This kind of complication, however, would rarely be worth pursuing for a mortality investigation and, in any case, forms part of the general subject of multiple decrements and is outside the present scope.

For a friendly society experience, there is less complication. New members join and old members withdraw from the society, and in some cases benefit ceases at certain ages so that members reaching such ages automatically become leavers.

For an experience of assured lives the leavers include lapses, surrenders for cash, possibly conversions to paid-up policy, if it is desired to exclude paid-up policies from the experience because of the difficulty in some cases of keeping in contact with the lives assured, and maturities by expiry of the endowment term. All of these could be treated as a combined group of leavers, but there are some practical complications. Nowadays, endowment policies usually mature at the end of a fixed integral number of years so that the assumption of a uniform distribution over calendar years and years of age is as valid at maturity as it is at entry. If maturity were, however, at a fixed age, such as 65, special treatment might be necessary, unless such cases formed only a small proportion of the whole group.

For the lapses, there are several practical features that require consideration. The general principle is clearly to take the lapses out of the exposed-to-risk from the moment that they leave the experience or, to put it another way, to include them as long as a claim would be paid on death. In practice, however, this principle cannot always be strictly followed, and various expedients have to be adopted. There is usually a short qualifying period before a policy acquires a surrender value, so that if a premium remains unpaid before the policy qualifies for a surrender value, it lapses. A policy of longer duration may, however, lapse first and be surrendered for cash after it has lapsed. Most premiums in ordinary life assurance are payable yearly, although a significant proportion are payable at half-yearly, quarterly or monthly intervals. Thus, uniformity of spread over years of duration might be an unsuitable assumption for the lapses. The position is further complicated by the fact that a period of grace is allowed for the payment of premiums. This is commonly 30 days, although it is often shorter for monthly premiums. For an experience in policy years a not unsuitable procedure that has been used is to take the duration for the lapses as the nearest complete number of years of duration, so that for yearly premiums the total duration of exposure from entry would be the same as the number of years' premiums paid despite the extra 30 days of 'life-assurance cover'. This would apply also for half-yearly and quarterly premiums where a complete number of years' premiums have been paid. An odd quarter's premium payment would thus not add to the total exposure, while two or three odd quarters' premiums and one odd half-year's premium would entail an extra year's exposure.

If the experience is based on enumerations of the policies in force on 1 January of successive years on the basis of the office's valuation records, the treatment for the exposed-to-risk would follow the view of its risks taken by the office for valuation purposes. The common practice is to include among the policies in force all those where the premium is still outstanding within the days of grace. The census formulae, and others based on census enumerations, thus automatically allow for the days of grace.

The position is, however, still further complicated by two further practical circumstances. First, there is the fact that lapsed policies are often revived on payment of the arrears of premium, possibly with an interest charge and revival fee. Then there is the practice of including in the policy conditions non-forfeiture clauses providing for policies which have acquired a surrender value to be kept in force for a period, which varies among offices, on the basis that the outstanding premium or premiums constitute an automatic loan on the security of the policy. This means that if death takes place the sum assured becomes payable subject to deduction of the arrears of premium which are also deducted if the policy is ultimately surrendered instead of becoming a claim.

Policies lapsing and reviving in the same year of observation would normally be treated as if they had been continuously in force. If the revival takes place in a later year than the lapse and each year's experience is being separately examined, the policy would be treated as a leaver in the year of lapse and as a new entrant (at the appropriate attained age and duration) in the year of revival. In an experience for a number of years combined it might be appropriate to ignore the lapse and revival altogether and to treat the policy as being continuously in force, particularly if most of the revivals have been allowed without any medical evidence of good health, either by reason of the operation of the non-forfeiture clause or because of a liberal office practice.

The treatment of policies kept in force under the non-forfeiture clause involves serious practical difficulties. To keep them all in the exposed-to-risk until the non-forfeiture period has expired may mean a departure from the office practice in its valuation which may be to carry a special overall reserve for such policies rather than to include them individually in the valuation. It may also mean keeping in the exposed-to-risk some policies which are completely lost sight of by the office because of the negligence of the policy-holder to keep in touch with the office or to enable the office to keep in touch with him. On the other hand, to exclude all policies while the non-forfeiture period is running does not permit all the corresponding deaths to be excluded because there is undoubtedly a strong tendency for such policies to be revived before death if the health of the life assured deteriorates during the non-forfeiture period, with the result that some deaths are included without all the corresponding policies being included in the exposed-to-risk. For the continuous assured lives' experience each calendar year's experience is, in essence, separately investigated, and offices are allowed latitude to deal with the non-forfeiture feature in the way which best suits their general office procedure. The consequence may be that the select mortality rates for some durations, par-ticularly for durations 2, 3 and 4, are somewhat inflated, with the result that the approach to the ultimate rates (i.e. rates for the same attained age but for the longer durations all combined) may appear to be more rapid than it really is. For the practical purposes for which the experience is investigated, however, the point is of little significance.

5·7. Combination of several years of experience

The combination of several years of experience with allowance for new entrants and leavers follows the same extended pattern as that described in the previous chapter with appropriate terms included for these extra items. This extended expression for the exposed-to-risk shows how the intermediate census enumerations cancel out and how the new entrants, leavers and deaths for the separate years combine together into one total each for each age. The process is illustrated for a 3-year period in the following state-ment for the exposed-to-risk at age $\{x\}$, where $\{x\}$ in the case of each symbol is the assumed age at the beginning of the year and the values of $_tP_{\{x\}}$ include all previous new entrants and exclude all previous leavers who have reached age $\{x\}$:

$$E_x = {}_0P_{\{x\}} + {}_1P_{\{x\}} + {}_2P_{\{x\}} + \tfrac{1}{2}n_{\{x\}} - \tfrac{1}{2}w_{\{x\}}$$
$$A + {}_0P_{\{x-1\}} - {}_1P_{\{x\}} + {}_0n_{\{x-1\}} - {}_0w_{\{x-1\}} - {}_0\theta_{\{x-1\}}$$
$$B + {}_1P_{\{x-1\}} - {}_2P_{\{x\}} + {}_1n_{\{x-1\}} - {}_1w_{\{x-1\}} - {}_1\theta_{\{x-1\}}$$
$$C + {}_2P_{\{x-1\}} - {}_3P_{\{x\}} + {}_2n_{\{x-1\}} - {}_2w_{\{x-1\}} - {}_2\theta_{\{x-1\}}$$
$$A + {}_0P_{\{x-2\}} - {}_1P_{\{x-1\}} + {}_0n_{\{x-2\}} - {}_0w_{\{x-2\}} - {}_0\theta_{\{x-2\}}$$
$$B + {}_1P_{\{x-2\}} - {}_2P_{\{x-1\}} + {}_1n_{\{x-2\}} - {}_1w_{\{x-2\}} - {}_1\theta_{\{x-2\}}$$
$$C + {}_2P_{\{x-2\}} - {}_3P_{\{x-1\}} + {}_2n_{\{x-2\}} - {}_2w_{\{x-2\}} - {}_2\theta_{\{x-2\}}$$
$$\vdots \qquad \vdots \qquad \vdots \qquad \vdots$$

down to and including the youngest age.

Therefore

$$E_x = \sum_{x-r}^{x} {}_0P_{\{x-r\}} - \sum_{x-r}^{x} {}_3P_{\{x-r\}} + \tfrac{1}{2}n_{\{x\}} + \sum_{x-r}^{x-1} n_{\{x-r\}}$$
$$- \tfrac{1}{2}w_{\{x\}} - \sum_{x-r}^{x-1} w_{\{x-r\}} - \sum_{x-r}^{x-1} \theta_{\{x-r\}}.$$

Writing b_{x-r} for $_0P_{\{x-r\}}$ and e_{x-r} for $_nP_{\{x-r\}}$ the exposed-to-risk for an n-year period can now be written down in the same form as in the previous chapter as follows:

$$E_x = \sum_{x-r}^{x} b_{x-r} - \sum_{x-r}^{x} e_{x-r} + \tfrac{1}{2}n_{\{x\}} + \sum_{x-r}^{x-1} n_{\{x-r\}}$$
$$- \tfrac{1}{2}w_{\{x\}} - \sum_{x-r}^{x-1} w_{\{x-r\}} - \sum_{x-r}^{x-1} \theta_{\{x-r\}}$$
$$= E_{x-1} + b_x - e_x + \tfrac{1}{2}(n_{\{x\}} + n_{\{x-1\}}) - \tfrac{1}{2}(w_{\{x\}} + w_{\{x-1\}}) - \theta_{\{x-1\}}$$

and
$$\mathring{q}_x \doteqdot \theta_{\{x\}}/E_x.$$

For the central rate the exposed-to-risk E_x^c is obtained by deducting $\tfrac{1}{2}\theta_{\{x\}}$ and allowing for the corresponding change from E_{x-1} to E_{x-1}^c on the right-hand side of the equation:

$$E_x^c = E_{x-1}^c + b_x - e_x + \tfrac{1}{2}(n_{\{x\}} + n_{\{x-1\}}) - \tfrac{1}{2}(w_{\{x\}} + w_{\{x-1\}}) - \tfrac{1}{2}(\theta_{\{x\}} + \theta_{\{x-1\}})$$

and
$$\mathring{m}_x \doteqdot \theta_{\{x\}}/E_x^c.$$

In the foregoing illustration of the combination of several years of experience it has been assumed that all the ages are strictly defined on the same basis at the beginning of each year so that the deaths, new entrants and leavers recorded at each age strictly correspond with the numbers living at the beginning and end of the relevant year.

In the last chapter (§4·3) we mentioned that the same principles apply when the deaths and the living are not in strict correspondence, and we showed how the discrepancies cancelled out subject to an adjustment for the last term in the summation of the deaths. Exactly similar considerations apply when the new entrants or leavers or both are not in strict correspondence with the living but detailed treatment of the exposed-to-risk formulae in such circumstances is deferred for consideration in Volume II.

5·8. The 'dynamic census' approach

In the last chapter we developed an arithmetical analogy with a multiple-decrement table by considering the number of lives l_x reaching exact age x while in the group at any time during the period of observation. This scheme can now be developed including provision for the new entrants and leavers. l_x thus includes all those who, before having attained age x, were in the group at the beginning or had entered the group during the period of observation, and had not left the group or died before attaining age x or were still in the group at the end of the period of observation at an age greater than x. We define the symbols b_x, e_x, n_x, w_x and θ_x to mean all the beginners, enders, new entrants, leavers and deaths at age x last birthday. Then

$$l_x = l_{x-1} + b_{x-1} + n_{x-1} - w_{x-1} - e_{x-1} - \theta_{x-1},$$

since those reaching age x must comprise all those reaching age $x-1$ plus the beginners and new entrants at age $x-1$ less the leavers, enders and deaths at age $x-1$.

By expressing l_{x-1} in terms of l_{x-2}, etc., l_{x-2} in terms of l_{x-3}, etc., and so on back to the youngest age, we can obtain l_x in Σ form as follows:

$$l_x = \sum_{x-r}^{x-1} (b_{x-r} + n_{x-r} - w_{x-r} - e_{x-r} - \theta_{x-r}).$$

By giving all the movements except the deaths half a year's exposure in the year of movement the exposed-to-risk for q_x is

$$E_x = l_x + \tfrac{1}{2}b_x + \tfrac{1}{2}n_x - \tfrac{1}{2}w_x - \tfrac{1}{2}e_x,$$

and

$$\mathring{q}_x \doteqdot \theta_x / E_x,$$

$$\mathring{m}_x \doteqdot \theta_x / (E_x - \tfrac{1}{2}\theta_x),$$

and

$$E_{x-\frac{1}{2}}^c = l_x,$$

$$\mathring{m}_{x-\frac{1}{2}} \doteqdot \tfrac{1}{2}(\theta_{x-1} + \theta_x)/l_x.$$

A similar process can be developed on the basis of all the ages being defined as nearest ages. In this case we should have

$$l_{x-\frac{1}{2}} = \sum_{x-r}^{x-1}(b_{x-r} + n_{x-r} - w_{x-r} - e_{x-r} - \theta_{x-r}),$$

$$E_{x-\frac{1}{2}} = l_{x-\frac{1}{2}} + \tfrac{1}{2}b_x + \tfrac{1}{2}n_x - \tfrac{1}{2}w_x - \tfrac{1}{2}e_x,$$

and

$$\mathring{q}_{x-\frac{1}{2}} \doteqdot \theta_x / E_{x-\frac{1}{2}},$$

$$\mathring{m}_{x-\frac{1}{2}} \doteqdot \theta_x / (E_{x-\frac{1}{2}} - \tfrac{1}{2}\theta_x).$$

5·9. The checking system with allowance for new entrants and leavers

The rough check on the exposed-to-risk computations indicated in §4·6 applies also when there are new entrants and leavers. We have again

$$\Sigma E_x \doteqdot \cdot 5n(\Sigma b_x + \Sigma e_x) + \cdot 5\Sigma\theta_x,$$

where n is the number of years in the experience. This approximate relation assumes that the new entrants, leavers and deaths are all uniformly spread over the whole period. To obtain a complete check the total new entrants, leavers and deaths should be totalled according to the year of observation in which they occurred. Thus

$$_tN = \sum_x {}_tn_x = \text{total new entrants in the } (t+1)\text{th year,}$$

$$_tW = \sum_x {}_tw_x = \text{total leavers in the } (t+1)\text{th year,}$$

$$_tD = \sum_x {}_t\theta_x = \text{total deaths in the } (t+1)\text{th year.}$$

The discrepancy between the left-hand side and the right-hand side of the above approximate checking relationship is exactly made up of

$$\sum_t [(t + \tfrac{1}{2} - \tfrac{1}{2}n)({}_tN - {}_tW - {}_tD)].$$

In practice, the figures for $_tN$, $_tW$ and $_tD$ may be readily available or readily ascertainable or there may be a record from which they can be approximately estimated. For example, the annual returns (A.R. 1) of a friendly society would be a useful source. The valuation records of a life office would usually provide a sufficient indication of the required figures. Some such checking process should always be carried through whenever possible. If for some reason one or other of the items making up the exposed-to-risk formula is based on some other approximation than a uniform spread over the year of observation so that some fraction of a year other than half a year has been used for the exposure in the year of movement, the relevant changes must of course be made in the checking process.

5·10. The 'dynamic census' approach for select rates

A similar approach can be used for select rates by defining $l_{[x]+t}$ as all those of entry age x who while in the group reached exact duration t at any time during the period of observation. By entry age is meant some uniform definition of age such as nearest age at entry, age next birthday at entry, age last birthday at entry and so on. Then $b_{[x]+t}$, $n_{[x]+t}$, $w_{[x]+t}$, $e_{[x]+t}$ and $\theta_{[x]+t}$ are defined according to entry age x and curtate duration t ($=$ completed number of years of duration). In general, $n_{[x]+t}$ would be the revivals at curtate duration t, but we need to distinguish the new entrants from the revivals at curtate duration o. We therefore write $n_{[x]}$ for the new entrants and $n_{[x]+0}$ for the revivals at curtate duration o.

Then

$$l_{[x]} = n_{[x]}$$
$$l_{[x]+1} = n_{[x]} + n_{[x]+0} + b_{[x]+0} - w_{[x]+0} - e_{[x]+0} - \theta_{[x]+0}$$
$$\vdots$$
$$l_{[x]+t} = l_{[x]+t-1} + n_{[x]+t-1} + b_{[x]+t-1} - w_{[x]+t-1} - e_{[x]+t-1} - \theta_{[x]+t-1}$$

and

$$E_{[x]+t} = l_{[x]+t} + \tfrac{1}{2} [n_{[x]+t} + b_{[x]+t} - w_{[x]+t} - e_{[x]+t}],$$
$$\hat{q}_{[x]+t} \doteqdot \theta_{[x]+t}/E_{[x]+t}.$$

As already indicated in the previous chapter, the 'dynamic census' approach will be considered more generally in Volume II.

5·11. The census method in practice

If new entrants and leavers are assumed to be uniformly spread over the year of age and over the calendar year we can still interpret $\frac{1}{2}({}_0P_x + {}_1P_x)$ as the mean population at age x last birthday throughout the calendar year. Thus all the formulae in § 4·8 make appropriate allowance for the new entrants and leavers (including migrants in a population experience) on the assumption of a uniform spread.

In a life office, year-end censuses of the policies in force are obtained by a continuous process. A system of obtaining year-end (valuation) ages is fixed. For example, the valuation age might be nearest age or age next birthday at entry plus curtate duration. Whatever system is used, the policies can be grouped into corresponding 'office years of birth'. For example, if the valuation year is N and the nearest age is x, the 'office year of birth' would be $N - x$ and a year later the valuation year would be $N + 1$, so that all those whose office year of birth is $N - x$ would have nearest ages $x + 1$ and so on. It is then a simple matter periodically to record all the new entrants, leavers and deaths in a given period (e.g. each month or each quarter or for a whole year) for each office year of birth and to maintain a running total of the number of policies in force for each group. Writing ${}_0P_{N-x} = {}_0P_{\{x\}}$ for the total in force at the end of one year for office year of birth $N - x$ and valuation age $\{x\}$ and n_{N-x}, w_{N-x} and θ_{N-x} for the corresponding movements in the ensuing year, we have

$$ {}_1P_{N-x} = {}_1P_{\{x+1\}} = {}_0P_{N-x} + n_{N-x} - w_{N-x} - \theta_{N-x} $$

for the number of policies in force at the end of the next year at valuation age $\{x+1\}$.

For office purposes, therefore, the valuation totals can be used as the basis for a mortality investigation, and this is in fact often done, particularly in industrial life assurance, although the census method of obtaining the rates of mortality is not usually employed. Instead, an exposed-to-risk formula is used which 'follows the lives through' the calendar year. Instead of taking

$$ \mathring{m}_{x-\frac{1}{2}} \doteqdot \frac{1}{2}(\theta_{\{x\}} + \theta_{\{x-1\}}/\frac{1}{2}({}_0P_{\{x\}} + {}_1P_{\{x\}}), $$

the formula often used is

$$ \mathring{m}_x \doteqdot \theta_{\{x\}}/\frac{1}{2}({}_0P_{\{x\}} + {}_1P_{\{x+1\}}). $$

For the Life Offices' continuous investigations the census formula is used, and for this the offices are required to tabulate the deaths, not according to the ages that they use in their valuation machinery, but according to nearest ages at death (or some other convenient approximation to exact age at death, on the average).

In practice, offices are not able to use their valuation totals for the continuous investigation because of the various policies that have to be excluded from the investigation. These include substandard lives, female lives, lives subject to occupational or residential extra premiums and concurrent duplicates (i.e. a policy effected within a short period of another on the same life in the same office which is included in the experience). However, by appropriately marking or punching the valuation cards applicable to policies included in the investigation, an 'investigation classification' can be continuously adjusted every time that the 'valuation classification' is adjusted, so that the investigation census totals can be scheduled for the mortality returns to the investigation committee. It is important to adjust the 'investigation classification' at the same time as the 'valuation classification' and not leave the movements to be totalled from the card files at the year-end because serious discrepancies can result if this is done. For example, consider a policy which stands lapsed at the beginning of the year (i.e. is not in the investigation census) and which revives and lapses again during the ensuing year. In the valuation system the card for this policy will first be extracted as a revival and then extracted as a lapse. It will thus be excluded from the year-end valuation census. It will, however, be among the file of cards of lapses for the year. If, therefore, the investigation adjustments are made from the year-end files this policy will be wrongly deducted from the previous year's census total.

CHAPTER 6

SICKNESS AND OTHER RATES

6·1. Preliminary considerations

For various reasons that we shall discuss, the idea of a sickness rate is more complicated and much less definite than the idea of a mortality rate. The complications and the vagueness are not, however, associated with the denominator of the rate. In fact, the principles of exposed-to-risk are exactly the same for sickness rates (or for any other kind of 'time-rate') as for mortality rates, although, as we shall see later, there are one or two technical points arising in connexion with sickness rates. It is with the idea of sickness itself as it affects the numerator of the rate that the main complications and special problems arise. There is nothing vague about the state of death or its alternative, survival. During a given period a person either dies or he does not; there is no middle condition. Sickness, on the other hand, is a relative idea. There are degrees of sickness, although there is not, of course, any obvious scale of measurement. It may be that, at a given time, some individuals can be definitely regarded as completely healthy (i.e. not sick), and, no doubt, others are just as definitely sick or ill. There would, however, usually be a middle group who for various reasons might or might not be regarded as sick according to the kind of definition and the strictness of the test of sickness adopted. We shall return to this question of definition later. Complications also arise out of the fact that sickness is not a simple once-for-all event; on the contrary, it is a continuing state which may terminate by death or by recovery. It may also recur in one form or another. For some purposes we might be interested in the proportion of persons in a given group who fell sick in a given period of time (e.g. a year), individuals falling sick more than once during the period being treated as single casualties. Such a proportion would, technically, be analogous to a mortality rate, since, on a suitable definition of 'falling sick' (which would usually include being sick at the

6   H & P

beginning of the period of observation), there would be only two mutually exclusive and exhaustive alternatives. If each bout of sickness were counted as a separate casualty this technical analogy with mortality rates would break down—for example, the sickness rate might in such circumstances exceed unity! No doubt, the analogy could be preserved by treating recoveries as new entrants for the exposed-to-risk, but for our present purpose we need not pursue this theoretical possibility. In whichever way successive bouts of sickness may be treated, a 'sickness rate' representing the proportion falling sick in a given period might have its interest and use as an ancillary statistic, but for most practical purposes something much more extensive, some measure not only of frequency but also of duration of sickness, would usually be required as well.

6·2. Two different forms of proportion sick

The idea of the proportion falling sick *during a period of time* should be sharply distinguished from the idea of the proportion sick *at a point of time*. The two ideas and the numerical values of the two proportions are quite different whatever period of time may be used for the former, although either can be used as a contributory factor in building up a 'durational' sickness rate of the kind used by actuaries for sickness insurance by the friendly societies and in National Insurance. In *Life and other Contingencies*, Volume I (p. 239), the idea of the proportion sick at a point of time is used to define sickness rates as used in actuarial work. We shall, therefore, first discuss the practical aspects of this idea before proceeding to the more direct approach commonly used in practical sickness insurance.

6·3. The proportion sick at a point of time and the definition of sickness

Let us suppose that for a given group of persons a sickness census is taken on a given day, a day being for practical purposes regarded as a 'point of time'. We should then want to know the total number of persons in the group and the total number sick. We should need some definition of 'sick'. A subjective definition (i.e. a definition based on the individual's personal judgment of his state of health) would be very unsatisfactory, because different people have very different ideas of when they are sick. We might use the definition 'being confined to the house' or 'being under doctor's orders', but some people are sick without being confined to the house and some consult a doctor much more readily than others. Further, what does 'being under doctor's orders' mean? Does it mean that a doctor has been seen that day or during the previous week or during the previous month? And, if it means one of these two latter ideas, how are we to deal with the idea of recovery since seeing the doctor and before the census date? If the group comprises only persons who are normally gainfully occupied we might define 'sick' as being away or retired from work by reason of sickness. But how are we to distinguish between the healthy unemployed and the unemployed who are sick? It is clear that the idea of sickness (or 'morbidity' as it is sometimes called) as a general sociological phenomenon is a very vague idea indeed. As an economic idea—absence from work through sickness—the phenomenon of sickness is not so vague, but precision of definition is still difficult to attain. The extent of the vagueness would usually be negligible for practical purposes if the group comprised, say, a group of employees in a particular organization or industry, provided that we do not inquire too closely into the possibilities of absenteeism and malingering.

Fortunately, for the purposes of actuarial statistics in relation to sickness insurance, whether under National Insurance or under private insurance as conducted by the friendly societies or the insurance companies, there is a relevant objective criterion which exactly fits the needs of the practical situation. If a claim to a day's sick pay has been successfully established the person concerned is treated as being sick for that day. The claim to sick pay is usually supported by a medical certificate and is sometimes checked by a special investigation of one kind or another. Whatever methods are employed for checking the validity of the sickness claims the resulting statistics are essentially statistics of the claims admitted rather than statistics of either objective or subjective sickness. Since one insurance organization may be more or less stringent in testing its claims than another, the claim statistics of the one may be quite unsuitable for use in connexion with the financial affairs of the other. Moreover, even when the statistics are analysed in ages or age-groups, the sickness experiences of different classes of persons (e.g. different occupational groups or residents in different regions) may vary considerably among themselves.

6·4. Definition of sickness rates in terms of the proportion sick

Let us now suppose that these difficulties have all been resolved and that we are able to record the total number in the group on a given day and the number who on that day are sick according to our definition (i.e. who are treated as absent from work through sickness or who have successfully claimed a day's sick pay), and let us suppose that we can take such a census for every working day during a given calendar year. If $_tP$ represents the number in the group at time t and $_tS$ represents the number sick at time t, then the proportion sick at time t, say $f(t)$, would be the ratio $_tS/_tP$. If it is assumed that there are no new entrants or leavers during the year and that $_tP$ is affected only by deaths, we may define the sickness rate for the calendar year either as $\sum_t {_tS}/_0P = \hat{s}$ (say) or in the 'central' form as $\sum_t {_tS}/(\sum_t {_tP}/N) = \overset{*}{z}$ (say), where N is the number of working days in the year on each of which a sickness census has been taken. Clearly $\sum_t {_tS}$ is the total number of working days lost during the year through sickness or the total number of days' sick pay successfully claimed for the year; $_0P$ is the number starting the year and is analogous to the exposed-to-risk for the q-type of mortality rate; $\sum_t {_tP}/N$ is the average total number in the group during the year (counting working days only) and is analogous to the exposed-to-risk for the m-type of mortality rate; $\hat{s}$ is the average number of days of sickness per person starting the year; and $\overset{*}{z}$ is the average number of days of sickness per person exposed during the year. For a 5-day working week $\hat{s}$ and $\overset{*}{z}$ would usually be divided by 5 and the result expressed in weeks. For a 6-day working week the divisor would be 6. For a $5\frac{1}{2}$-day working week it would seem that the Saturday morning or other half-day should be treated as a half-day's exposure and a half-day's sickness. In practice, however, both in National Insurance and private insurance, the half-day is usually treated as a full day and the week treated as a 6-day working week. If the group is a large one in which there have been a number of deaths spread fairly uniformly over the year the expression $\left(_0P - \dfrac{\sum\limits_t {}_tP}{N}\right)$ would be approximately equal to half the deaths for the year. Hence we may write

$$\tfrac{1}{2}\mathring{q} \doteqdot (1 - \tfrac{1}{2}\mathring{p}) \doteqdot \left(1 - \frac{\sum\limits_t {}_tP}{_0PN}\right),$$

and since

$$\mathring{s} = \mathring{z} \times \sum_t {}_tP/(_0P \times N),$$

$$\mathring{s} \doteqdot \tfrac{1}{2}\mathring{p}.\mathring{z}.$$

6.5. Idealization of the sickness rate

If we idealize $_tP$ and $f(t)$ by assuming that they each vary continuously throughout the year, the sickness rate $\mathring{z}$ expressed in terms of a year as the unit of time, is then

$$\frac{\displaystyle\int_0^1 f(t).{}_tP\,dt}{\displaystyle\int_0^1 {}_tP\,dt},$$

and this may be compared with the definition of the theoretical central sickness rate at age x given in *Life and other Contingencies* (p. 240) as follows:

$$z_x = \frac{52.18 \displaystyle\int_0^1 f_{x+t}l_{x+t}\,dt}{\displaystyle\int_0^1 l_{x+t}\,dt},$$

where l_{x+t} is the life-table function and the factor 52.18, representing the average number of weeks in a year, changes the measurement of the sickness from years to weeks.

6·6. The total sickness in the year

The idealized expression $\int_0^1 f(t) . {}_tP\, dt$ represents the total sickness in years during the year, and it may be compared with

$$\sum_t {}_tS = \sum_t f(t) . {}_tP,$$

which represents the actual total sickness in the year expressed in working days. It may thus be seen that for the sickness rate the daily censuses are required only to build up the figure for the total sickness in the year. The denominator of the central rate, i.e. the central exposed-to-risk, can be obtained in the usual way by deducting half the number of deaths in the year from the number starting the year. If, therefore, the total sickness can be obtained in a simpler way the daily censuses can be dispensed with. In fact, such a simpler approach has long been in use by actuaries for friendly society and other sickness insurance statistics. This approach is to record in respect of each individual the number of weeks and odd days of sickness in the year and to compute the total of such weeks and days for the group, taking care to convert every 6 days (or 5 in the case of a 5-day week) into a week.

A simple arithmetical variant of this procedure is to compute the average period of sickness for all those who are sick during the year and to multiply the average by the proportion falling sick during the year. If we write F for the proportion falling sick during the year we have the identity

$$\hat{s} = F \times \sum_t {}_tS/(F_0P) = \sum_t {}_tS/{}_0P.$$

In practical actuarial work it is sometimes helpful to consider these two component factors of $\hat{s}$ separately. The second factor of $\hat{s}$ itself comprises two factors: (a) the average number of spells of sickness per person falling sick and (b) the average duration per spell. If there is no linking up of spells of sickness for the same individual the sickness rate may factorize in the form $[F.(a)] \times (b)$ instead of in the form $F \times [(a).(b)]$ as given above.

6·7. The frequency distribution of durations of sickness

When compiling the statistics of total sickness reference has usually to be made to the duration of sickness of each individual. As we are concerned only with sickness in the investigation year the duration of sickness of any individuals who were sick at the beginning of the year would be computed on the assumption that their sickness began then; similarly, for those still sick at the end of the investigation year their sickness would be assumed to terminate at the year-end. If the information is on cards, a convenient way of doing the work would be to sort the cards according to the number of days' sickness suffered by the individual and then to tabulate the number of individuals for each number of days' sickness. A simple computation would then provide the total sickness. Even if a more direct method of obtaining the total sickness is available (e.g. from punched cards), the tabulation of the frequency distribution of durations of sickness would be a simple process and would be well worth doing for the insight that it provides into the incidence of sickness as between sickness of short, medium and long duration. It has the further theoretical advantage that it enables an estimate of the standard deviation of the sickness rate to be made for the purpose of judging the significance of variations in the rates from time to time and between different groups. If $_0P$ represents the total number in the group at the beginning of the year and n_i represents the number having i working days of sickness in the year—n_0 being the number with no sickness—then

$$n_0 + n_1 + n_2 + \ldots = \sum_i n_i = {_0P},$$

$$F = \text{the proportion sick} = ({_0P} - n_0)/{_0P},$$

and
$$\bar{i} = \hat{s} = \sum_i i n_i / {_0P},$$

where s is the ordinary sickness rate referred to the number starting the year. If we wanted z we should need to know the deaths θ in order to arrive at the central exposed-to-risk. Thus

$$\hat{z} \doteqdot \sum_i i n_i / ({_0P} - \tfrac{1}{2}\theta).$$

The second moment of the n_i distribution about the origin o is

$$\sum_i i^2 n_i /_0 P,$$

and the second moment about the mean is

$$\mu_2 = \sigma^2 = \sum_i i^2 n_i /_0 P - (\sum_i i n_i /_0 P)^2.$$

By using the observed value of σ^2 as the estimate of the variance and applying the usual formula for the standard deviation of a mean, $\sigma_m = \sigma \cdot {}_0 P^{-\frac{1}{2}}$, we obtain for the standard deviation of $\hat{s}$

$$\sigma_s^2 \doteqdot {}_0 P^{-2}[\sum_i i^2 n_i - (\sum_i i n_i)^2 /_0 P].$$

The approximate variance of the total sickness can be written in the form

$$\sum_i i n_i [\sum_i i^2 n_i / \sum_i i n_i - \sum_i i n_i /_0 P].$$

Since all those who are not sick contribute nothing to the moments about the origin o, we can write the approximate variance in the following alternative form:

$$\text{total sickness} \times \left(\frac{m_2}{m_1} - F \cdot m_1\right),$$

where m_1 and m_2 are the first and second moments about o of the sickness durations of all those who are sick (i.e. excluding those who are not sick) and F is the proportion sick. Since $m_2 > m_1^2$ and provided that F is not too large, we might further approximate by omitting the second term within the brackets, viz.

$$\sigma_S^2 \doteqdot \text{total sickness } (m_2/m_1).$$

Since the moments m_1 and m_2 could be estimated sufficiently closely from a random sample of claims (possibly at quinary or denary age-intervals when sickness rates are analysed by age) to provide an approximation to the value of m_2/m_1 at successive ages, it will be seen that an approximate significance measure is obtainable from the claims alone without computing the exposed-to-risk. This result may be compared with the approximation, based on the Poisson law, for the standard deviation of the deaths, given by the square root of the deaths instead of the binomial value $\sqrt{(Epq)}$.

G. F. Hardy in 1888 devised the approximate formula $2\sqrt{S}$ for the mean deviation of the sickness. Assuming that the mean deviation is ·8 of the standard deviation the corresponding approximation to the variance is

$$\sigma_S^2 \doteqdot 6{\cdot}25S,$$

where S and σ are expressed in 6-day weeks. σ^2 in days is, of course, $6^2 \times (\sigma^2 \text{ in weeks})$, and S in days is $6 \times (S \text{ in weeks})$, so that Hardy's formula in days becomes

$$\sigma_S^2 \doteqdot 37{\cdot}5S.$$

Thus Hardy's formula takes $37{\cdot}5$ as an approximation for

$$(m_2/m_1 - F.m_1).$$

The accuracy of this approximation depends on the shape of the sickness distribution. Evidently, the distribution is highly skew with a long tail towards the longer periods of sickness. For the diminishing exponential distribution ($n_i \propto e^{-im_1}$) we have $m_2 \doteqdot 2m_1^2$, while for the diminishing triangular distribution ($n_i \propto 3m_1 - i$) we have

$$m_2 \doteqdot 3m_1^2/2.$$

In the Manchester Unity experience the value of F for 'all sickness' of the A.H.J. Group was ·213 at age 25, ·216 at age 35, 241 at age 45, ·297 at age 55 and ·434 at age 65, with rapidly growing proportions at the older ages. Thus, if we exclude the older ages, the value of σ_S^2/S for the Manchester Unity A.H.J. experience was probably in the neighbourhood of $1{\cdot}25m_1$. The values of m_1 were 24, 29, 41, 65 and 113 days for ages 25, 35, 45, 55 and 65 respectively. Hardy's approximation of $37{\cdot}5$ is, therefore, only a very rough average figure, but it would serve to provide a rough indication of significance limits for a large experience on the basis of two or three standard deviations on either side of the mean, provided that it was not applied at the older ages or to the partial sickness statistics for the individual pay-periods.

6·8. Periods of reduced sick pay and the off-period

In sickness insurance, particularly as conducted by friendly societies, it is usual to provide, in respect of each sickness attack, for the rate of benefit to be reduced after a fixed duration of sickness and to be further reduced after further fixed durations of sickness. For example, there might be a reduction to half-pay after 3 months and to quarter-pay after 6 months. In applying the rules governing these reductions it is usual to link up all claims not separated by a minimum off-period (commonly taken as a year) and to treat a succession of linked-up claims as a single continuous period of sickness. Sickness attacks separated by more than the off-period are treated as distinct attacks for the purpose of determining the rate of benefit.

The system of reduction of the rate of sick pay makes it essential to separate the total sickness and the sickness rates into the various 'periods of sickness' if the statistics are to be used for financial purposes. If all the members were 'off the funds' at the beginning of the investigation year and no attacks of sickness occurred subsequently which required to be linked up with a previous attack before the beginning of the investigation year, statistics in the form of the frequency distribution of durations of sickness discussed in §6·7 would provide all that was needed for subdivision of the sickness according to rate of sick pay. This, unfortunately, is not so, and for each individual the situation calls for two measures of sickness duration, i.e. the duration of sickness in the investigation year, (i) and the linked-up duration (j) which determines the rate of sick pay at the commencement of the sickness in the investigation year. As an alternative to recording j we might record $l\ (=i+j)$, the linked-up duration at the end of the sickness in the investigation year, and for some purposes this might be a preferable course, i and l both then being durations at the termination of the sickness. A bivariate frequency distribution according to i and j or i and l would clearly enable the total sickness to be divided up either in the ranges of linked-up durations corresponding to the rates of sick-pay or according to shorter ranges for use in a variety of problems. The classic Manchester Unity Experience 1893/97 provided for each age x five convenient sickness duration ranges, viz. first 3 months, second 3 months, second 6 months, second 12 months and after 2 years. Sickness 'after 12 months' and 'after 2 years' arises, of course, because of the linking up, for rate-of-pay purposes, of sickness that occurred in the years immediately preceding the investigation year. G. F. Hardy subsequently devised an approximate technique for splitting up the rates at each age (see §6·10 for the analysis of sickness rates by age) into individual weeks, a process that could have been easily done from the data if the bivariate frequency distribution had been recorded for each age. L. E. Coward (*J.I.A.* **75**, 12) has shown how to use detailed sickness rates of this kind to estimate the variance of the sickness rates, but the analysis is too intricate for reproduction here.

In day-to-day actuarial work when the sickness experience of a society is investigated for the purpose only of the finances of the particular society the simple procedure would be used of recording separately the number of weeks and days of sickness which rank for full pay, reduced pay, further reduced pay and so on. Writing S_1, S_2, S_3, etc., for the total sickness eligible for full pay, reduced pay, further reduced pay, etc., and $\mathring{s}_1, \mathring{s}_2, \mathring{s}_3$, etc., for the corresponding rates, we then have the following additive relation:

$$\mathring{s} = S/_0P = S_1/_0P + S_2/_0P + S_3/_0P + \text{etc.},$$
$$= \mathring{s}_1 + \mathring{s}_2 + \mathring{s}_3 + \text{etc.},$$

i.e. the sum of the partial rates equals the all-sickness rate.

The expression in §6·7 for the standard deviation of $\mathring{s}$ applies also to each of the partial sickness rates provided that we interpret n_i as the number of members successfully claiming for i days' sickness at the relevant rate of pay.

6·9. Influence of reductions of sick pay on sickness rates

From time to time statistical evidence has been produced (e.g. A. W. Watson, *J.I.A.* **62**, 29) showing that the reduction of the rate of sick pay has an influence on the rate of recovery or, more realistically, on the rate of return to work. The extent of this phenomenon depends upon the degree of efficiency of the administration of claims as well as upon the economic factor as it affects the individual. However, the point serves to stress that sickness in the statistical sense is significantly under human control. It also serves to stress the dangers of assuming without investigation that sickness statistics obtained from one organization are suitable for use in connexion with another organization whose arrangements may be significantly different in their impact upon the decision to go 'sick' or to remain 'sick'.

6·10. Sickness rates analysed by age

So far we have discussed the problems of compiling sickness rates for a group of persons over a calendar year. Total sickness rates show a marked tendency to rise with age in much the same way as mortality rates, although the partial rates may show a different or less definite trend. Subdivision of the group by age is, therefore, usually necessary if a proper view of the experience is to be obtained. The problem of allocating the exposed-to-risk over the ages is the same as for mortality rates. The allocation of the sickness to the individual ages also follows the same principles as for the deaths. The sickness for a given age should normally be that relating to the lives included in the exposed-to-risk at that age, so that if the ages for the exposed-to-risk are defined as at the beginning of the calendar year the sickness should be allocated by reference to the age at the beginning of the calendar year. The principle of correspondence applies, but if a similar latitude with regard to approximate correspondence such as is possible in a mortality experience is taken, a complication arises in the allocation of the sickness to the individual ages. For example, if the exposed-to-risk are according to nearest age on 1 January and the sickness is to be according to age last birthday at the date of the sickness, in many cases the sickness in the calendar year would have to be divided between two adjacent ages. It might be, for example, that some first-period sickness and part of some second-period sickness would be allocated to age x and the rest of the second-period sickness to age $x+1$. For this reason it is usual to preserve a strict correspondence between the sickness and the exposed-to-risk.

It would, of course, be possible to make a life-year investigation or a membership-year investigation, but as sickness investigations are, in practice, almost invariably on a calendar-year basis, we shall not pursue these possibilities.

The process of combining two or more years of experience follows the same lines as for a mortality investigation, the exposed-to-risk being combined in exactly the same way and the sickness at each age being combined in the same way as the deaths. Continuous exposed-to-risk formulae equally apply to a sickness investigation.

6·11. New entrants and leavers

A feature sometimes found in the rules of a friendly society is the provision that no sick pay will be allowed for sickness in the first n months of membership. This period, which may be 6 months, is usually called the 'waiting period'. The obvious course to take would be to defer the inclusion of new entrants in the exposed-to-risk until n months after the date of entry. In practice, however, the new entrants are often recorded according to their actual years of entry and ages at entry, and accordingly appropriate adjustments have to be made for the exposed-to-risk. Apart from this point the fractional exposure to be allowed for new entrants follows the same lines as for a mortality investigation.

A common feature affecting sickness benefits is a rule providing for complete cessation of benefit on reaching a fixed advanced age such as 65 or 70 or on retirement. These cases are appropriately dealt with as leavers by providing for the fractional exposure in the year of cessation on the same lines as for the leavers in a mortality investigation. Members may, however, cease paying contributions before reaching the maximum age. The rules may provide for the defaulting members to continue in full benefit for a fixed period (e.g. 6 months) and then to go out of benefit for a period (e.g. another 6 months) before being finally struck off the membership roll. A member who puts himself back into benefit by paying up his arrears of contribution would be treated as having been continuously in benefit. Any attempt to allow for the hiatus in eligibility for benefit would be fraught with difficulty and would not usually be justified by the effect on the results. Some kind of health test —at least a declaration of good health—would usually be required to prevent defaulting members from getting back into benefit while sick merely by paying up the arrears. Adjustments are, however, usually made for members actually struck off the roll. The easiest course would be to ante-date the date of leaving to correspond with the date of going out of benefit, but in practice these leavers are often recorded in the year in which, and at the age at which, they are struck off the roll, and appropriate adjustments have to be made in obtaining the exposed-to-risk similar to those required in respect of the waiting period for the new entrants.

When an investigation is being made into the sickness experience of a large friendly order in which the rules or practice may differ among the lodges some reasonable practical rule must be adopted for dealing with the new entrants and leavers. It was this feature of variation between the lodges that created the need for the special treatment accorded to new entrants and leavers in the Manchester Unity Experience 1893/97. An example of the kind of adjustments made is given in §6·12.

6·12. An illustration of a sickness investigation

Let us suppose that an investigation is to be conducted into the sickness experience in the 5 years 1949–53 of a society granting sickness benefits in the form of full pay for the first 6 months, half-pay for the next 6 months and quarter-pay thereafter, subject to a 1-year off-period, a 6-months' waiting period and a 3-months' out-of-benefit period before expulsion. The data would be collected on cards, either hand-written or punched. These cards would normally be completed by the officials of the society. A suitable form of hand-written card is illustrated in Table 6·1.

TABLE 6·1

Front	Back

| No....... Name..............
 Occupation .... Sex......
 Date of birth ....
 Date of entry......... Age......
 Date of exit .... Age......
 Cause of exit ....
 Other information..............
 ....
 .... |

		Sickness Claims			
			Period		
Year	Age	1st	2nd	3rd	
		W D	W D	W D	
1949					
1950					
1951					
1952					
1953					
Total					

In filling in the particulars of the sickness, reference may be made to the rate of pay actually paid in order to allocate the sickness to the correct periods. The actual amount paid at each rate could be recorded instead of the number of weeks and days, and the total amounts at each age for each rate of pay could then be converted into weeks by dividing by the appropriate rate of pay. If only the dates of the sickness are recorded in the society's records it would be necessary to refer all cases of sickness in the first year of the investigation back to the sickness in the preceding year or two in order to secure a proper allocation of the sickness to the appropriate periods having regard to the provision for linking up separate periods of sickness under the off-period rule. Sometimes this course would be dispensed with except for members actually claiming at the commencement of the period of the investigation.

The form in which to take the age would depend on the information available. Often the date of birth would not be available. The year of birth might be available, in which case the age last birthday on 1 January could be used for all members. Alternatively, the only information available about age might be the age next birthday at entry, in which case the age on 1 January would be taken as age next birthday at entry plus the curtate duration. Let us assume that age last birthday on 1 January of each year is available for all members and that new entrants and leavers have been recorded according to their actual dates of joining and leaving and not according to the dates of coming into and going out of benefit. In these circumstances, of course, the details on the cards would take a somewhat different form from that indicated in the specimen card shown above.

We now define

b_x as the beginners at age x last birthday on 1 January 1949;

e_x as the enders at age x last birthday on 1 January 1954;

n_x, w_x, θ_x as the new entrants, leavers and deaths during the period of the investigation whose age last birthday on 1 January of the calendar year of entry, leaving or death was x; (it is assumed that all the leavers are expulsions).

$S_x^{m/n}$ represents the total number of weeks of sickness in the pay-period 'n weeks after m weeks' during the period of the investigation in a calendar year in which the age of the life on 1 January was x.

We have now to decide on the appropriate adjustments for the new entrants and leavers. A simple course for the new entrants would be to exclude them entirely from exposure at the age corresponding to the calendar year of entry, and to give them a full year's exposure at the age corresponding to the year following the year of entry. The justification for this course would lie in the balancing of a deficit of exposure in the calendar year of entry with an excess of exposure in the following year. The entrants in the first half of a calendar year may be suitably regarded as exposed, on the average, for a quarter of a year in the year of entry on the usual uniformity assumptions; the entrants in the second half are not exposed at all; while the entrants in the second half of the previous year should be exposed in the year following their year of entry for only three-quarters of the year on the average. To carry out this process we should need to know the number of new entrants in the half-year next before the commencement of the period of the investigation which are included in b_x. Instead, therefore, of including in the exposure at age x in the calendar year t the items $\frac{7}{8} \times {}_{t-1}n_{x-1} + \frac{1}{8} \times {}_t n_x$, the simple course that would usually be adopted in practice in the circumstances envisaged in which there is a 6-months' waiting period, would be to give ${}_{t-1}n_{x-1}$ a full year's exposure at age x in year t and not to expose ${}_t n_x$ at all at age x in year t.

Similar arguments apply for the leavers. Those occurring in the last 9 months of a calendar year would, on the average, be exposed for $\frac{3}{8}$ of the year, while those in the first 3 months of the year would not be exposed at all in that year and on the average would have been exposed in the previous year for only $\frac{7}{8}$ of that year. To make allowances on these lines we should need to know the leavers in the first 3 months after the end of the investigation period which would have been included in e_x. For the exposed-to-risk at age x in year t we ought therefore to deduct $(\frac{1}{4} + \frac{3}{4} \times \frac{5}{8})_t w_x = \frac{23}{32}{}_t w_x$ and also $(\frac{1}{4} \times \frac{1}{8})_{t+1} w_{x+1}$. The practical course, instead of this, would be to deduct $\frac{24}{32}{}_t w_x = \frac{3}{4}{}_t w_x$.

The continuous exposed-to-risk formulae (x = age last birthday) would then be as follows:

$$E_x = E_{x-1} + b_x - e_x - \theta_{x-1} + n_{x-1} - \tfrac{3}{4}w_x - \tfrac{1}{4}w_{x-1},$$
$$E_x^c = E_x - \tfrac{1}{2}\theta_x,$$
$$s_x^{m/n} = S_x^{m/n}/E_x,$$
$$z_x^{m/n} = S_x^{m/n}/E_x^c.$$

These rates are for ages last birthday, since the ages are all defined as ages last birthday on 1 January. The same formulae would apply if the ages were all defined as age x nearest birthday on 1 January and the rates would then be for nearest ages.

6·13. Standard tables

The only sickness investigation for which full details have been published and which has formed the basis of an extensive set of standard tables is the Manchester Unity investigation of 1893–97. The Manchester Unity standard tables, with or without adjustment, are still in use today for friendly society work, and the report on the investigation may still be profitably studied at first hand for its practical as well as its theoretical interest; only a brief summary will, however, be given here.

The Manchester Unity of Oddfellows comprises a large number of lodges spread throughout the Kingdom, each lodge having a large element of autonomy in its administration, its rules and its finance. One of the main objects of the investigation was to provide a large volume of actual sickness and mortality data which could be used to form the basis of a number of standard tables from which to choose the most suitable for the valuation and other purposes of particular lodges. We have already mentioned the need to adopt uniform assumptions to deal with various waiting periods and withdrawal rules. These assumptions were different for mortality and sickness. A uniform off-period of 12 months was used to link up the sickness, and sickness rates for the uniform periods mentioned in §6·8 were computed despite the variation in the rules governing rates of pay in the different lodges.

The mortality and sickness data were divided between three

major geographical areas of residence, and each of these groups was subdivided into rural and urban areas according to density of population and further subdivided according to eight broad occupational groups. After a careful analysis and study of the results it was decided for the purpose in view to construct separate mortality tables from the data of each of the geographical areas, taking the rural and urban data separately and together. For the sickness tables the occupations were grouped into three broad groups. It is the table of sickness rates for one of these groups (the A.H.J. table) that is still largely in use in conjunction with more modern mortality tables.

The reader should not conclude from the decisions taken with regard to the groupings of the data for the construction of standard tables that it was thought that the only environmental factor affecting mortality was geographical area of residence and that occupation was the only important factor for sickness rates. The decisions were convenient for the practical purposes in view and took account of the fact that individual lodges tended to be dominated by a particular occupation which was often fairly widespread in the district in which the lodge operated. It was, therefore, not unreasonable to use tables for a particular lodge based on the sickness of the dominant occupation and the mortality of the district.

6·14. Durational effects on sickness rates

While it is not usual for a friendly society to require a new entrant to submit to medical examination, it is usual to exclude persons who are already sick and to endeavour to exclude impaired lives by such means as requiring applicants to sign a declaration of good health. As a consequence some element of 'selection', i.e. lighter sickness at the same age for recent entrants than for earlier entrants, should be exhibited by the all-sickness rates. The use of a waiting period seems, therefore, to be unnecessary, but while it serves as a further safeguard against the admission of poor lives, it also reduces the significance of 'selection' due to the initial health requirements. In fact, no account is usually taken in friendly society work of this kind of selection. There is, indeed, a much more significant durational effect which also is usually ignored in the broad treatment that is commonly sufficient for the financial problems of friendly societies. This durational effect is shown in the changing incidence of sickness in the separate pay periods which from the very nature of the case must persist for a good many years. The point can be most simply explained by reference to one or two examples. A new entrant obviously cannot possibly claim in the first year in the pay period 'after 12 months', nor in the second year in the pay period 'after 2 years'. For a group of new entrants a number of years must elapse before, as a group, they become liable to the full force of the later-period rates applicable to members of the same age who have been in the society for a longer period. In the meantime the early-period rates of the recent entrants may be abnormally high, unless the all-sickness rates are sufficiently low owing to the initial health selection. In the Manchester Unity investigation members of different durations at the same attained age were grouped together, and 'average' partial rates were computed despite the disturbance due to the practice of admitting new entrants up to quite advanced ages such as 40 or 45. In connexion with 'transfer values' under National Health Insurance, as it was operated before the National Insurance Act 1946 abolished the Approved Society system, this inherent 'selection' was regarded as an important factor. A member transferring from one Approved Society to another was necessarily a non-claiming member. Accordingly, for the purpose of computing the transfer value to be passed from the one society to the other, a set of adjustments to the sickness rates on which the National Health Insurance finances were based was devised. Full details are given in a paper by P. N. Harvey (*J.I.A.* **54**, 150).

6·15. Problems arising out of special rules affecting sickness benefits

Among the many friendly societies in existence there are all kinds of variations in the rules affecting sickness benefits, quite apart from the variations in the length of the waiting period and of the off-period. Sometimes the rules are designed to restrict payments due to long attacks of sickness, regarding the function of the society as providing benefits for short-term sickness rather than for permanent disability. Sometimes the rules are designed merely to keep the claims within the scope of a modest rate of contribution. Any investigation into the experience of a society with the view to providing a financial basis for the operations of the society must necessarily be concerned with successful claims to benefit rather than with sickness as such. A member who, although sick, is not entitled under the rules to benefit would be treated in the investigation as 'not sick'. Actuaries are thus concerned with claim rates rather than with sickness rates.

Sometimes the effect of the rules is to render unsuitable the usual assumptions regarding the uniform distribution of sickness over calendar years or years of age, thus requiring special treatment for the leavers. As an example, we may mention an actual case where members were entitled to not more than 8 weeks' sick pay in any one calendar year. Clearly the usual treatment of leavers would be unsatisfactory because a member might leave early in a calendar year after drawing all or most of his current maximum sick pay for 8 weeks. The actual procedure would depend on the circumstances, including the significance of the withdrawal rate and we cannot discuss the question *in vacuo*.

A fairly common type of limitation of benefit is for continuous sickness benefit to be restricted to, say, 6 months at a time. After receiving sick pay for 6 months the member would be ineligible for a period fixed by the rules, e.g. for a year. He would then become eligible again for benefit. The year of ineligibility should not be confused with the off-period which might also operate if there is more than one rate of pay. A member who is permanently disabled would receive benefit in a recurring cycle. The cycle might, for example, be full pay for 6 months, half pay for 6 months, no pay for a year, full pay for 6 months and so on.

The usual principles apply for the purpose of computing the sickness claim rates, but difficulties may arise when it is desired to compare the rates with those of some other society or with a standard table or to modify the rates of a standard table as a basis for valuation. Valuation procedure in such cases is discussed in *Friendly Societies* by W. T. C. Blake and J. M. Moore.

6·16. Withdrawal rates

In a pension fund, benefits are often payable on withdrawal from the fund and withdrawals occur continually. Even for non-contributory funds in which there is usually no benefit on withdrawal, the element of withdrawal may be allowed for in the financial basis of the fund. Whether this is so or not, statistical information regarding the incidence of withdrawals will usually be required in conjunction with the investigations made preliminary to the periodical valuation of the fund. Withdrawal is like death, in that it operates to remove the member from the membership. If the benefits on withdrawal and death were the same we might combine them and obtain the total decremental rates. The investigation would then be just like a mortality investigation except that the rates would be for 'death or withdrawal', i.e. in the notation used in *Life and Other Contingencies* for multiple-decrement rates we should have

$$a\hat{q}_x^{d \text{ or } w} \doteqdot (\theta_x + w_x)/E_x^{d \text{ or } w},$$

where E would be computed by exposing the deaths and the withdrawals up to the end of the 'year' of death or withdrawal. This total decremental rate could be split into its component parts

$$a\hat{q}_x^d \doteqdot \theta_x/E_x^{d \text{ or } w}$$

and

$$a\hat{q}_x^w \doteqdot w_x/E_x^{d \text{ or } w}.$$

These partial rates are, in principle, similar to the partial sickness rates of the s-type although sickness is not, of course, a decremental phenomenon. An even better analogy would be with partial death-rates analysed according to some classification of causes of death. Let us suppose that groups (a), (b), (c), etc., of causes of death have been defined. Then

$$\hat{q}_x \doteqdot \theta_x/E_x = \theta_x^a/E_x + \theta_x^b/E_x + \theta_x^c/E_x + \text{etc.}$$

Returning to the discussion of withdrawal rates, we might prefer to obtain the total central rate, viz.

$$a\hat{m}_x^{d \text{ or } w} \doteqdot (\theta_x + w_x)/E_x^c \doteqdot (\theta_x + w_x)/(E_x^{d \text{ or } w} - \tfrac{1}{2}\theta_x - \tfrac{1}{2}w_x).$$

The partial central rates would be

$$a\mathring{m}_x^d \doteq \theta_x/E_x^c,$$

$$a\mathring{m}_x^w \doteq w_x/E_x^c.$$

It will be observed that while $a\mathring{m}_x^d$ is identical with the usual central death-rate $\mathring{m}_x$ and $a\mathring{m}_x^w$ is defined in an identical way, the partial death-rate $a\mathring{q}_x^d$ differs from $\mathring{q}_x$ because in the former the withdrawals are exposed up to the end of the year of withdrawal, while in the latter the withdrawals are exposed only up to the date of withdrawal on the average. We could define a withdrawal rate in a form identical with $\mathring{q}_x$ by giving the withdrawals a full year's exposure in the year of withdrawal and the deaths only half a year's exposure in the year of death. Using the symbol $\mathring{q}_x^w$ for such a rate we have the third analogous pair of rates

$$\mathring{q}_x \doteq \theta_x/E_x^d \doteq \theta_x/(E_x^{d \text{ or } w} - \tfrac{1}{2}w_x),$$

$$\mathring{q}_x^w \doteq w_x/E_x^w \doteq w_x/(E_x^{d \text{ or } w} - \tfrac{1}{2}\theta_x).$$

Unlike the partial rates and the central rates, these 'single-decrement' rates have different expressions for their exposed-to-risk corresponding to the treatment of 'the other decrement' as an extraneous decrement for which an adjustment of the exposed-to-risk is required.

These three pairs of rates provide examples of the three different approaches to the problem of multiple-decrement tables which will be taken up in Volume II.

Lapse rates are sometimes required in connexion with life-assurance policies. The principles are exactly the same as for withdrawal rates as discussed above except that select rates in durations of assurance would usually be required in view of the greater prevalence of lapses at the shorter durations. In practice, lapses would not be uniformly distributed over the policy years owing to the mode of payment of the premiums, e.g. an annual-premium policy can lapse only at the end of the days of grace following the due-date of the premium. Lapses would, however, include surrenders for cash and conversions to free policy which might occur at any time in the policy-year. Revivals would usually be treated as negative lapses, and their number at a given age and duration would be deducted from the corresponding number of lapses. Net lapse rates of the form $\bar{q}^{w}_{[x]+t}$ would usually be computed.

6·17. Retirement rates

The provisions for retirement on pension vary considerably from one pension fund to another, but there is often an option available to members to retire on pension at any time between a minimum and a maximum age, e.g. from 60 to 65. Current practice in framing rules often provides nowadays for a fixed normal pension age with provision for early or late retirement, and no doubt late retirement will be more common in the years to come in view of the growing proportion of the aged to the total population. In computing retirement rates in ages a concentration of retirements at particular age-points may need special treatment. The kind of thing that may happen is that a definite proportion of those reaching, say, aged 60 retire on or near their 60th birthdays; then there may be a steady flow of retirements with possibly minor concentrations at the 61st to 64th birthdays with the remainder retiring on their 65th birthdays. In such circumstances the exposed-to-risk must take account of the practical features. The number retiring at age 60 in the investigation period would be related to the total number reaching age 60 in the period to produce a 'point-rate' at age 60. A similar process would be used for retirements at age 65. For intermediate retirements the usual yearly type of rates would probably be appropriate. In practice it would often be sufficient to compute rates for the retirements between ages 60 and $60\frac{1}{2}$, between $60\frac{1}{2}$ and $61\frac{1}{2}$ and so on up to $64\frac{1}{2}$ to 65.

6·18. Incapacity retirements

Many pension funds provide for a pension benefit to commence on retirement as a result of an accident or a breakdown in health causing 'total permanent' incapacity to continue working. Accordingly, an investigation into the rates of incapacity retirement is often required as well as the mortality and withdrawal investigations. The principles are the same as for the other decrements and we have a choice of a 'total-decrement' rate comprising three partial rates, or of three central rates, or of three separate single-decrement rates. If the membership is large enough, it may be worth while to investigate the mortality of the incapacity pensioners separately. This would be done in select form showing the rates according to age at retirement and duration since retirement. Investigations of this kind have shown rates of mortality which are very heavy immediately after retirement, falling fairly rapidly over about 5 years and then merging into an ultimate table of rates somewhat higher than the normal mortality rates for the same age. Provision may be made for the pension to cease on recovery of health, but these cases are usually too few to make an investigation of the incidence of recovery worth while.

Similar problems arise in connexion with what is called 'permanent disability' insurance which is much more common on the Continent of Europe and in America than in the United Kingdom. The actuarial principles employed involve the rates of becoming disabled and the rates of mortality and recovery among the disabled. The more liberal the office is in judging disability claims the greater becomes the premium that is necessary for the risk, the greater the need to pursue the possibilities of recovery and the more nearly the insurance approaches to a sickness insurance of the kind granted by friendly societies. It is a moot point at what stage in the range between a full sickness insurance and a strict total permanent disablement income insurance it is wise to pass from the sickness technique to the technique of rates of occurrence and rates of recovery, but this question is beyond the scope of this book.

6·19. Marriage rates and fertility rates

For actuarial financial purposes marriage and fertility, or issue, rates are of little significance because, apart from state insurance and certain small marginal benefits in certain friendly societies, these events are not usually the subject of monetary benefits. The main reason for this situation is that these events are largely under the control of the individual and are, therefore, unsuitable subjects for commercial insurance. They are, however, of great importance in demographic studies. Marriage and fertility rates are rarely computed for longer periods than a year, and few special problems arise with regard to the exposed-to-risk. The technical problems arising are mainly concerned with the subdivision of the data, the manipulation of the available data to serve particular statistical purposes and the interpretation of the results. The levels of marriage and fertility rates are both influenced by changing economic and political conditions. Marriage rates may be obtained in the form of a percentage of the marriages to the total males (or females) in each subgroup or to the number of unmarried males (or females) in the subgroup. Similarly, fertility rates may be expressed in terms of all women (or men) in the subgroup or in terms of all married women (or men) only—there are various complications to be dealt with, such as illegitimate births, still-births, multiple births and the related question of the difference between maternities and births. The proportion married in each subgroup provides the link between rates based on the married and rates based on the married and unmarried combined, but whichever of the two forms of rates are recorded or even if, as is better, both are recorded the problems of interpretation are difficult. Marriage rates inevitably depend on the supply of suitable partners of the other sex—a point of special significance in a period following a war or heavy migration—and high rates at one time tend to generate low rates later on as the supply of both partners diminishes. Marriage rates of both sexes vary greatly with age as well as with various other characteristics, such as social class, occupation, area of residence and so on. Widowhood, divorce and remarriage complicate the statistical problems. Fertility rates depend partly on the level of marriage rates in the recent past, and this applies to fertility rates in terms of the married only as well as to those in terms of the married and unmarried combined. They also vary greatly with age, duration since marriage and the number of previous children—a woman who has had a maternity cannot, of course, have another for a period of nearly 12 months.

There is a considerable element of interaction between marriage and fertility rates from time to time and between different subgroups. For various practical purposes actuaries combine together sets of mortality rates to form mortality tables and also sickness rates and withdrawal and retirement rates to form hypothetical models similar in nature to the mortality table. The legitimacy of this procedure depends upon the practical purpose to be served. Owing to the interactions and the secular changes in the level of the rates, to construct similar tables based on marriage and fertility rates without reference to any particular practical problem is a highly dangerous statistical procedure and is likely to lead to false conclusions about the course of these phenomena in the actual population from which the rates were compiled.

For further information about marriage and fertility statistics the reader is referred to *Demography* by P. R. Cox.

CHAPTER 7

THE PRINCIPLES OF GRADUATION AND THE GRAPHIC METHOD

7·1. Introduction

So far we have been mainly concerned with various processes of obtaining rates of mortality or sickness or other rates for a succession of ages, or durations, from the experience of a group of lives over a period of one or more calendar years. In an orderly development of our subject we might at this stage proceed in one of two different directions. We might proceed to consider the various ways that have been devised from time to time of manipulating the observed rates or the data upon which they are based, with the view to making comparisons with the rates of other experiences or with some given table or tables of rates. This part of our subject has, however, been fully treated in Chapter 7 of Cox's *Demography*. Accordingly, we shall not discuss comparative methods—including mortality indices—except to the extent to which particular comparative processes may be incidental to the other parts of our subject; for this purpose we shall include a brief *ad hoc* discussion to avoid assuming that the reader is familiar with the relevant parts of *Demography*.

7·2. The purposes of graduation

We can, therefore, proceed at once in the alternative direction of development which is to discuss the principles and methods of the process long known by the label 'graduation'. In the course of time this label has been both extended and narrowed in its application, according to the particular interests of various writers. For example, the process of manipulating a succession of sets of mortality rates for a particular group of lives (e.g. the male population of England and Wales) over successive periods of time with the view to projection into the future might be embraced in the word 'graduation'. On the other hand, some aspects of the testing of a graduation might be included within the ambit of the theory of testing of statistical hypotheses, while the actual process of graduating the observed rates might be a subject for a general philosophical discussion on the function of hypotheses in scientific method and on the various ways in which hypotheses are set up. Our present purpose, however, is much more mundane and practical, and these wider implications of 'graduation' will not be discussed. Our concern is principally with the principles and methods of adjusting a set of observed rates to provide a suitable basis for actuarial calculations in connexion with various practical problems. In fact, our interest will be still further narrowed because we shall take a static view of the phenomenon that is the subject of our set of rates. For example, we shall assume that mortality is not changing with time. It would, of course, be more realistic to state this assumption in the form that it is sufficient for our practical purposes to assume that mortality is not changing with time. In this form, however, the relatively meticulous processes of graduation become inappropriate because the needs of the practical situation would then be fully met by a hypothetical set of mortality rates differing from the observed rates by much more than would usually be tolerated in a set of graduated rates. The effect also of the economic factor in practical actuarial work is such as to render inappropriate a meticulous approach to the statistical basis; most actuarial problems require assumptions regarding future interest rates as well as future mortality or other statistical rates. The result is that from a strictly practical point of view graduation has come to be regarded as an unnecessarily refined technique and we should not dissent from this view. Nevertheless, the principles of graduation are of basic importance to a proper appraisal of the behaviour of actuarial statistics and to the development of a sound judgment in the selection of a statistical basis for practical problems and the testing of such basis by experience.

7·3. The justification for graduation

The fundamental justification for the graduation of a set of mortality rates is the assumption, suggested by experience, that if the number of individuals in the group on whose experience the statistics are based had been much larger, the set of observed rates would have shown a much more regular progression from age to age (or from duration to duration) and that, in the limit, if the number in the group had been indefinitely large the set of rates might well have exhibited the kind of smooth progression that we are accustomed to see in the tabulated values of the more usual kinds of mathematical function. As we mentioned in Chapter 1 'smoothness' is a difficult concept to define mathematically, and it is a fact that not all mathematical functions exhibit what we instinctively regard as smoothness; indeed, mathematical functions can be defined to exhibit the very opposite of smoothness. No attempt will be made to give even a working, let alone a rigorous, definition of smoothness. Instead, we shall adopt the customary pragmatic approach of testing for an undefined smoothness by examining the second and third differences of the graduated statistics to see whether they are small—or, if not small, whether they in their turn progress smoothly!

Instead of contemplating that our group might have been indefinitely large in number we might compare the rates applicable to the same group for successive calendar years. Unfortunately, apart from the possibility of a time trend in the rates, it is a fact of observation that substantial differences in mortality, extending over long ranges of ages, occur between successive calendar years due to differences in general prevailing conditions of which the effect of the weather is perhaps the most important in the short run. As another alternative we might consider what the position might have been if we could have observed an 'identically similar' group in 'identically similar' circumstances. The phrase 'identically similar' is vague, but it is not intended to rule out random differences, particularly in the statistical outcome of the run of the rates. The logical difficulty involved in this vagueness touches the very foundations of the philosophy of science and we pass hurriedly on.

The point we want to make is our expectation based on experience that a 'similar' group in 'similar' circumstances would exhibit a set of rates broadly 'similar' to the original set in general level and general progression from age to age but with roughnesses of progression showing no pattern of similarity with the roughness of progression of the original set. In fact, we should expect the roughnesses to have the character of 'randomness'. This is another vague undefined concept whose practical manifestations we usually have little difficulty in recognizing, although mathematical statisticians have in recent years developed various more or less rigorous processes for testing for its existence in practical data.

7·4. Random error and 'intrinsic' roughness

To avoid the practical and theoretical difficulty involved in observing a second group of lives 'similar' to the first we might divide our actual group of lives into two equal subgroups by some completely unbiased random process such as writing a slip for each life—whether a survivor or a death—and putting all the slips in a well-shuffled heap and then drawing a slip alternately for each of the two subgroups. The differences in the statistical outcomes, i.e. the differences between the sets of mortality rates shown by the two subgroups, would, however, merely reflect the random process of the drawing, and we are no nearer to a justification for our expectations regarding the nature of the roughnesses in our observed set of rates. Nevertheless, we can see from this illustration that the roughnesses might be of two totally different kinds. They might be due (1) to what we may call 'intrinsic' roughnesses, or sharp changes in the course of the rates, which have nothing whatever to do with chance or randomness and (2) to random variations whose incidence from age to age we should not expect to be repeated if the experience itself could be repeated. The presence or otherwise of 'intrinsic' roughnesses is usually determinable, from a practical point of view, from our general knowledge of the circumstances of the group of lives and from the knowledge of the progression of the rates of mortality of other groups of lives of not widely dissimilar constitution and in not widely dissimilar circumstances of environment and period of observation.

7·5. Circumstances in which 'intrinsic' roughnesses may be removed

When 'intrinsic' roughnesses exist in a set of rates the answer to the question of whether they should be smoothed out by a graduation process would depend on the knowledge available concerning the reasons for their existence and on the purpose which the graduation is to serve. If it is to produce a statistical basis for actuarial calculations relating to the future and if, as would usually be the position, the reasons for the 'intrinsic' roughnesses were not thought likely to persist or to be of any practical importance, the obvious course would be to remove them in the process of graduation. But then their removal would need to be kept in mind and fully allowed for when testing the graduation for 'goodness of fit' (see *Statistics* by Johnson and Tetley, Vol. II, Chapter 17). It is possible to apply tests to a set of observed rates to ascertain whether the general level of roughnesses can be fully explained by random variations without the need to assume the existence of 'intrinsic' roughnesses, and this is, of course, a great help in setting a standard for a test of 'goodness of fit'. We need not pursue this aspect here beyond mentioning that a full discussion of one such test devised by Michaelson and Redington is contained in R. H. Daw's paper entitled 'On the validity of statistical tests of the graduation of a mortality table' (*J.I.A.* **72**, 174). If the purpose of a graduation is merely to exhibit the experienced rates with the random roughnesses removed or at least reduced, a graduation process should be adopted which avoids smoothing out the 'intrinsic' roughnesses, and the resulting 'graduated' rates would not, therefore, be expected to exhibit complete smoothness. An example of this kind is provided by the methods used for the English Life Tables where the aim is to preserve the 'inherent' features of the experience as far as possible. These methods are discussed in the next chapter.

For the rest of the discussion we shall assume that our data do not exhibit any 'intrinsic' roughnesses or at least that, in so far as 'intrinsic' roughnesses exist in the data, their removal by the graduation process is not undesired.

7·6. Smoothness and fidelity to the data

With the foregoing preliminary discussion in mind the immediate object of a graduation process may be expressed variously as a smoothing process or as a process of removing roughnesses or as a process of removing or reducing random errors. This reference to reducing random errors does not imply any hypothesis regarding their statistical distribution. For the process of graduation itself no such hypothesis is really needed; it is only at the stage of testing a graduation that a distribution hypothesis may be needed. Regarding graduation as a smoothing process leads to the idea that the most satisfactory graduation of a particular set of statistics would be that one which while securing the desired degree of smoothness departed as little as possible from the original statistics. Thus for comparing two or more graduations we need not only to test each of them for smoothness but also for fidelity to the original data, or, in Karl Pearson's phrase, for 'goodness of fit'. It is obvious that complete fidelity would mean no smoothing whatever and that perfect smoothness would mean at least a certain amount of departure from the original data. Thus it has sometimes been stressed that smoothness and fidelity are conflicting objectives in graduation and that some optimum compromise is required. While this is a correct statement as far as it goes, it seems better to regard graduation in the first place as the elimination or reduction of random errors which inevitably leads to smoothness unless the data are subject to 'intrinsic' roughnesses. It is only if there are 'intrinsic' roughnesses to be removed by graduation that we need to think of smoothness and fidelity as in conflict, that is, when we are making *systematic* departures from the observed statistics.

7·7. Methods of graduation

There are three broad categories into which the processes of graduation may be divided. They are as follows:

(1) Graphical methods in which 'smoothness' is achieved by drawing on graph paper a curve that runs through the main path of a set of points representing the observed data. The curve may be drawn freehand or with mechanical aids.

TABLE 7·1

x	u_x	e_x	v_x	u'_x	e'_x	v'_x
1	10	+1	11	—	—	—
2	16	−3	13	—	—	—
3	23	+2	25	24	+·2	24·2
4	31	+1	32	32	−·4	31·6
5	40	0	40	41	0	41·0
6	50	−2	48	51	+·2	51·2
7	61	−1	60	62	−·2	61·8
8	73	+3	76	74	+·4	74·4
9	86	−1	85	—	—	—
10	100	+3	103	—	—	—

(2) Finite-difference methods, including what are known as 'summation formulae'. These methods depend upon the principle that the standard error of the weighted mean of two or more independent (or imperfectly correlated) random errors is less than the sum of the correspondingly weighted individual standard errors, e.g. if a set of random errors e_i are independent of each other, we have

$$\sigma_m^2 = \Sigma w_i^2 \delta_{e_i}^2 < (\Sigma w_i \sigma_{e_i})^2,$$

where $m = \Sigma w_i e_i$ and $\Sigma w_i = 1$.

Thus if we operate upon a set of observed values by a process of moving averages, the process partially eliminates the random errors, which may be positive or negative, by averaging them. The weights in this case would, of course, be equal. Unfortunately, the moving-averages process operates also upon the 'basic' values as well as upon the random errors—in practice, of course, the two are not separately given—and if the 'basic' values are not linear a systematic error is introduced. The process also reduces any 'intrinsic' roughness in the data in much the same way as it reduces the random errors. A simple example will bring out the points more clearly than any amount of verbal description. In Table 7·1 the basic values u_x are parabolic and the random errors e_x are arbitrary. The 'graduated' values $v'_x = u'_x + e'_x$ represent the effect of using a simple five-year moving-average process on the 'observed' values, $v_x = u_x + e_x$. This process, of course, gives the same

8

values of v'_x as would be obtained by operating on u_x and e_x separately and then adding the two results together. The systematic error in this case, $u' - u$, is exactly unity at each value of x for which a graduated value can be obtained.

Various refinements of the moving-average process have been devised, which in principle all reduce to substituting for v_{x_1} a weighted average of v_x for various values of x surrounding x_1. These refinements are directed to selecting the weights, including negative weights, so that the systematic errors are reduced to unimportant dimensions and so that the general level of the residual random errors e'_x is as small as possible consistent with their smooth progression.

(3) Curve-fitting methods. These methods depend upon the assumption that the 'basic' values take a particular mathematical form which may be selected for theoretical reasons or merely for empirical reasons, depending upon the knowledge of the general shape and trend of the set of observed values to be graduated. The mathematical formula selected would usually contain a number of parameters for which numerical values need to be fixed to secure a 'good fit'. The various processes of finding suitable values for the parameters can be considered from the point of view of various optimum principles that have been set up in mathematical statistics, but, in practice, refinements of fitting techniques are not often worth pursuing.

7·8. Distribution of grouped data

Closely associated with graduation are the various processes of distributing data grouped for ranges of the independent variable (e.g. quinary age-groups) over the individual values of the variable (e.g. over individual ages) and of interpolating graduated values between pivotal values given at intervals of the independent variable. These processes may also be carried out by graphical, finite-difference or curve-fitting methods.

Attention will now be confined to graphical methods of graduation, distribution and interpolation. Summation methods of graduation will be treated in Volume II. Finite-difference methods of distribution and interpolation will be treated in the next chapter. Curve-fitting methods are treated in Chapter 17 of Volume II of Johnson and Tetley's *Statistics*.

7·9. Graduation of exposed-to-risk and deaths separately

In principle, whatever method of graduation is to be used we have a choice of working either with the exposed-to-risk and the numbers of deaths (or other events) separately or with the corresponding set of rates directly. There is usually, however, little to be gained by doing two graduations instead of one, and the assumption of basic underlying smoothness of the two series of numbers comprising the exposed-to-risk and deaths is much more likely to be inappropriate than the corresponding assumption for the rates. It is possible for the rates to be free from any significant degree of 'intrinsic' roughness in circumstances in which the exposed-to-risk and deaths show quite sharp changes from age to age. In such a case the practical objections to operating on the exposed-to-risk and deaths separately would be strengthened. Nevertheless, in such circumstances it might be practicable, if for any reason it were so desired, to graduate the exposed-to-risk in such a way as to smooth out the sharp changes by making the graduated curve cut through them and then to make a recomputation of the deaths for graduation purposes by multiplying the graduated values of the exposed-to-risk by the observed rates of mortality. Indeed, this course may be desirable in any case when operating on the numerators and denominators of the rates separately, otherwise a slightly different treatment of waves or abrupt changes in progression for the deaths from that accorded to the exposed-to-risk might well result in the rates obtained by division from the two graduations showing irregularities which would require a further smoothing process for their removal.

In graduating the exposed-to-risk and deaths separately by any method it is necessary to decide first whether the two series of numbers are to be regarded as point-functions of the age at discrete unit intervals or as equivalent to areas on a succession of unit bases. For example, if E_x is the exposed-to-risk based on nearest ages and θ_x is the number of deaths at age x last birthday, we can either

(i) graph E_x (and θ_x) as a succession of ordinates proportional to E_x (and θ_x) erected at unit intervals on the x-axis and then draw a smooth curve as closely as possible to the tops of the ordinates, sometimes passing above and sometimes below, but without any particular bias one way or the other—the graduated values would then be obtained by reading off the heights of the ordinates of the smooth curve corresponding to the integral ages: or

(ii) graph E_x (and θ_x) as a histogram in the form of a succession of rectangles with areas proportionate to E_x (and θ_x) on unit bases from $x - \frac{1}{2}$ to $x + \frac{1}{2}$ (from x to $x + 1$ for θ_x) and then draw a smooth curve as closely and as fairly as possible through the tops of the rectangles—the graduated values would then be obtained by assessing the areas enclosed by the base line, each pair of successive ordinates and the corresponding arc of the smooth curve.

7·10. Graphical distribution of grouped totals

In practice, if E_x and θ_x are graphed for each individual age, there is little difference between the ordinate and the area procedure because the mid-points of the tops of the rectangles of the histograms can be treated as the tops of a succession of ordinates. If, however, an element of interpolation is required as well as graduation, e.g. if E_x and θ_x are given in 3-year group-totals and graduated values at unit intervals are required, then the area procedure comes into its own, in application as well as in principle. In such a case the histograms would be obtained by graphing each group-total as a rectangle with area equal to the group-total and with base equal to the age-range of the group. When the smooth curves have been drawn the graduated values are represented by the relevant areas on unit bases.

Even when E_x and θ_x are given at unit intervals it may sometimes be helpful—particularly if the data are not very numerous—to combine them into group-totals and then to draw the histograms. The age-ranges of the group-totals might well be arbitrarily selected. They need not be the same for E_x and θ_x, and successive age-ranges may be unequal as long as care is taken to make each rectangular area of the histograms conform to the total in the group. The choice of age-ranges for the grouping would be made by trial to achieve as fair a run as possible of the average values of E_x and θ_x in each group before proceeding to the work of graphing. This process assists considerably in showing how to draw a fair smooth curve through the tops of the rectangles.

7·11. Irregularities in population totals at successive ages

One of the earliest mortality tables to be constructed, the Carlisle Table, was produced by graphing as histograms the group totals of the mean populations and deaths that were given in quinary age-ranges up to age 20 and in denary age-ranges thereafter. The primary purpose of the procedure was obviously to distribute the group-totals over the individual ages, and accordingly the 'smooth' curves that were drawn through the tops of the group-total rectangles show some curious twists and turns. These were, presumably, embodied in the graduated curves because there was some ancillary information which suggested that the numbers at successive ages did not run steadily downwards as does the l_x column of a mortality table. This absence of any real justification for assuming that P_x and θ_x should show a regular progression from age to age is emphasized by consideration of the present age-distribution of the population of Great Britain with all its twists and curls due to sharp changes in the numbers of births in successive years in the past, to the incidence of the age and time distribution of migrations in the past and to the effects of the casualties of two world wars in which arbitrary age-limits for the call-up were adopted from time to time. Some of these disturbances are today much more marked than the disturbances due to age-errors and the preference for final digits such as 0, 2 and 5 in the statements of age. These age-errors were once quite marked, but with improved education and the more meticulous requirements with regard to age for National Insurance purposes systematic age-errors at the census are nowadays much less extensive.

It will often be found that the set of values of E_x for an experience extending over a number of years has a quite remarkable regularity. This results from the automatic smoothing effect of the summation processes used in obtaining E_x from b_x, n_x, etc. Each of these component items is itself a frequency distribution with its own general shape and 'intrinsic' and random irregularities. For example, n_x and w_x represent the age distributions of new entrants and leavers in the period of observation. Each life entering into E_x must be either a beginner or a new entrant. If all the b_x lives were exposed throughout the n years of the experience they would each be included in E_x at each age x to $x+n-1$ inclusive. The effect would be exactly the same as taking n times the n-year moving average of b_x. Of course, some of the beginners die or leave during the period, but a large part of the smoothing effect nevertheless remains. The same effect in less degree applies also to the new entrants. In general, an ogive $F(x) = \Sigma^x f(x)$, formed from a frequency distribution $f(x)$, is 'smoother' than the frequency distribution itself —E_x is, of course, a combination of ogives. There are two reasons for this greater smoothness. First, in summing to form the ogive irregularities or 'errors' of different sign tend to cancel each other out. Secondly, the net resultant 'error' in $F(x)$, i.e. $\Sigma^x \delta_x$, is in general a much smaller proportion of $F(x)$ than the individual 'error' δ_x is of $f(x)$. Roughness, or absence of smoothness, is essentially a relative characteristic.

7·12. Graphical estimate of μ_x from populations and deaths

Sometimes it is useful to graph E_x^c and θ_x as areas in the form of histograms and then to read off the ordinates at unit age-intervals. This might be particularly suitable if, for some purpose, we desired to make estimates of μ_x at, say, quinary intervals. The justification for this lies in the following two assumptions, namely, that

$$E_x^c = \int_0^1 l_{x+s}\,ds$$

and
$$\theta_x = \int_0^1 \mu_{x+s} l_{x+s}\,ds + \text{a random error.}$$

If the data were given in, say, quinary age-groupings, these integrals would extend over 5 years. We can now see that the histogram rectangles can be regarded as representing these integrals and that the 'smooth' curves can be regarded as representing the functions

$$l_{x+s} \quad \text{and} \quad \mu_{x+s} l_{x+s},$$

so that the ratio of their values for particular values of s can be taken as estimates of μ_{x+s}. The smoothing process, if successful, has, of course, reduced the effect of the random errors.

7·13. Graduation of rates directly

The process of graduating the exposed-to-risk and deaths separately, as a means of obtaining a set of graduated mortality rates is not free from practical difficulty, particularly if adjustments of the graphs have to be made to remove awkward features in the graduated rates such as can arise from the division of two sets of numbers which are not entirely free from roughnesses. This process is not likely to be used in practice, therefore, unless some special purpose is to be served thereby. If the sole object of the work is to produce a set of graduated rates the more practical course would usually be to operate directly upon the rates themselves.

If a set of points on a graph representing the observed rates of mortality at successive ages of a group of adult lives are joined together by straight lines, we obtain a typical jagged line with a fairly clear underlying trend that is so characteristic of the graphs of various kinds of observed statistics, particularly those shown by economic time-series. The jaggedness comes from the irregularities —'intrinsic' and random—that are superimposed upon the underlying trend line that is usually assumed to be relatively smooth. It is this smooth trend line that it is the function of graduation to reveal. In the case of mortality rates the size of the irregularities—the amplitude of the jaggedness—necessarily depends upon the size of the exposed-to-risk. In a really large experience the graph of the rates might well show only a relatively small degree of roughness, and the drawing of the appropriate smooth curve representing the general sweep of the rates would be fairly simple although a certain amount of adjustment and polishing might be necessary before the result would be considered satisfactory. In drawing the curve all unnecessary curvature, waves and inflexions in the curve would be avoided. What is unnecessary in this respect is a matter for judgment in the light of our general knowledge of the run of other sets of mortality rates and of the results of testing the graduation curve for smoothness and 'goodness of fit'—tests of graduation are discussed in §7·15. It is possible to form a general view of the degree of roughness and of the size of the irregularities to be removed before graphing the rates. By differencing the rates and examining the size and signs of the differences we can see at once the extent of the roughness—large first differences and frequent changes of sign are obvious indications of roughness.

The graduation problem is thus to draw a smooth curve following the general run of the jagged path of the observed rates, i.e. to draw a curve running between the observed points instead of through them so that graduated rates may be read from the graph. It is, of course, usually desired that the smooth curve should not be 'unfair', that is, that it should not in general show greater or smaller rates than the observed rates either over short stretches of age or over the whole age-range, although for some practical purposes a bias in one direction may be preferable to a bias in the other. In judging whether there has been a bias in either direction it is necessary to bear in mind what is usually known as 'the weight of the data'. If, for example, the rate at age x is based on an E_x which is considerably more than the E_{x-1} and E_{x+1} upon which the rates at ages $x-1$ and $x+1$ are based, more influence would normally be accorded to $\mathring{q}_x$ than to $\mathring{q}_{x-1}$ and $\mathring{q}_{x+1}$ in deciding where to draw the graduation curve. In practice, however, as we saw in §7·11 E_x usually runs fairly regularly from age to age, and this question of 'weight' is, therefore, usually not of much significance over short stretches. But it may be of considerable importance in relation to the graduation as a whole. Usually in the middle age-ranges the data are much more extensive than they are at the extremes. Thus while the graduation curve may be relatively easy to draw in the middle range where the amplitude of the swings in the graph of the observed rates may be relatively small, the reverse is the position at the extremes where the amplitude may be very large indeed if the data are very few. There are two ways of coping with this difficulty. The first is to bring to our aid our general knowledge of the size and general run of the mortality rates of other experiences at those ages which may be extreme for our particular experience but not for the others. For example, ages below about 55 would be 'extreme' for an annuitants' experience but not for an experience of assured lives. At the oldest ages the data are always few in number, but here we usually rely upon the assumption—it is only an assumption—that mortality rates continue to increase towards unity in extreme old age. Precision in the rates at the oldest ages is, however, rarely if ever of any significance from a practical point of view.

The other way of coping with the difficulty of large swings in the observed rates is to make a judicious combination of the data for short ranges of ages and to graph the corresponding group-rates as rates for the age approximately corresponding to the centre of gravity of the set of values of E_x included in the group. In practice, it is usually sufficient to take the mid-point of the age-range of the group as the centre of gravity. If the observed rates, apart from irregularities, show any significant degree of curvature even the centre of gravity as the age corresponding to the group-rate would impart a bias, but over short age-ranges this is rarely of any significance in comparison with the size of the irregularities that need to be removed by graduation. These points about the centre of gravity and curvature need, however, to be kept in mind for the occasional awkward case where they are of more than usual significance.

In fixing the ages to be grouped a certain amount of experimentation may be desirable. The ranges of the groups need not, of course, be equal. In fact, it is a help in securing a preliminary reduction of irregularity to use unequal groups. On the other hand, fixed arbitrary age-groups may often be good enough and may help in avoiding the temptation to draw the smooth curve too closely to the observed group-points. It is worth bearing in mind that, on the usual binomial assumption, the standard deviation of the number of deaths corresponding to ΣE_x over a short range of ages closely approximates to $\sqrt{(\Sigma E_x \hat{q}_x)}$ (i.e. the square root of the total actual deaths at the ages in the group) provided that the number of deaths in the age-group is not too small. Thus, for any particular group-point taken in isolation, the smooth curve might quite well pass as far away from the observed group-rate as corresponds to two standard deviations of the deaths on an approximate confidence-interval basis at the 1 in 20 confidence level. If, however, unequal groupings have been adopted to reduce the irregularities as much as possible the criterion of two standard deviations becomes inappropriate for judging isolated groups. The reason for this is that the process of selecting the age-ranges involves a deliberate offsetting of 'errors', and so there is an artificial correlation introduced which reduces the standard errors. But this does not justify going to the other extreme and running the smooth curve either through or too near to the group-points. It is precisely this fault—amounting to 'undergraduation'—that is apparent in T. B. Sprague's graphic graduation of the mortality experience of the Government Female Annuitants (1884) (excluding the first 4 years after purchase) described in detail in his classic paper on Graphic Graduation (*J.I.A.* **26**, 77, 1886) which remains the standard work on the subject to this day. The mortality rates shown by the experience used by Sprague for his illustration strike us today as somewhat strange. They start at about $17\frac{1}{2}$ per thousand in the early twenties, fall to about 10 per thousand in the early thirties and then rise steadily up to nearly 50 per thousand at age 70, apart from a very shallow depression which Sprague allows in the graduated rates commencing at about age 40 and reaching its nadir in the mid-forties—possibly due to his views on the effects of childbirth and the change of life. Nowadays the corresponding rates would start at less than 2 per thousand at age 20 and rise steadily up to about 25 per thousand at age 70 and 180 per thousand at age 90. With such a range of variation it would be very desirable to break the graduation work into at least two and preferably three overlapping sections, using different scales for the three sectional graphs as may be convenient for obtaining graduated rates to the required number of significant figures. The sections should sufficiently overlap to ensure a satisfactory junction between them.

Although Sprague's data are so much out-of-date and give rates so unlike the rates of a modern experience, it is useful to use a section of his example to illustrate the preceding discussion. Accordingly, in Table 7·2 are set out for the ages 45–61 the values of E_x, θ_x and $\mathring{q}_x$, and the data for his third trial groupings which he adopted for his actual graduation. Sprague did his graphical work

TABLE 7·2. *Government Annuitants' Experience* (1884)—*female lives, excluding the first 4 years after the purchase. Exposed-to-risk, numbers of deaths and observed rates of mortality. Ages 45–61 only*

Age x	E_x	θ_x	$1000\mathring{q}_x$	Age x	E_x	θ_x	$1000\mathring{q}_x$
45	1252	17	14	54	3330	59	18
46	1416	21	15	55	3682	57	15
47	1578	13	8	56	4104	83	20
48	1761	14	8	57	4473	86	19
49	1958	26	13	58	4885	90	18
50	2160	22	10	59	5281	123	23
51	2387	37	16	60	5644	138	24
52	2669	43	16	61	6038	116	19
53	2909	51	18				

Age-group	Central age	Group E	Group θ	Group $1000\mathring{q}$
45–51	48	12,512	150	12·0
52–55	53·5	12,590	210	16·7
56–58	57	13,462	259	19·2
59–61	60	16,963	377	22·2

TABLE 7·3. *Sprague's graduated rates as read from the graph in Fig. 7·1 and the corresponding differences and deviations*

Age x	Graduated $1000q_x$	$1000 \times \Delta q_x$	$1000 \times \Delta^2 q_x$	$1000 \times (\mathring{q}_x - q_x)$	$E_x q_x$	Actual deaths minus $E_x q_x$
45	11·3	—	·1	3	14·2	2·8
46	11·3	·1	—	4	16·0	5·0
47	11·4	·1	·5	−3	18·0	−5·0
48	11·5	·6	·3	−4	20·3	−6·3
49	12·1	·9	·1	1	23·7	2·3
50	13·0	1·0	·5	−3	28·1	−6·1
51	14·0	1·5	−·7	2	33·4	3·6
52	15·5	·8	−·1	1	41·4	1·6
53	16·3	·7	—	2	47·4	3·6
54	17·0	·7	—	1	56·6	2·4
55	17·7	·7	—	−3	65·2	−8·2
56	18·4	·7	·1	2	75·5	7·5
57	19·1	·8	·1	0	85·4	·6
58	19·9	·9	·2	−2	97·2	−7·2
59	20·8	1·1	·2	2	109·8	13·2
60	21·9	1·3	—	2	123·6	14·4
61	23·2	—	—	−4	140·1	−24·1

in three sections. The selection of the age-range 45–61 which extends over the junction of two of these sections is therefore unfair to Sprague but it is useful for the present illustrative purposes. In Fig. 7·1 the observed rates for these ages, the corresponding group-rates and the graduation curve that he drew are recorded. In Table 7·3 Sprague's graduated rates are recorded together with their first and second differences and the deviations between the actual and graduated rates. A further brief reference is made to these results in §7·16 after the subject of testing graduations has been discussed.

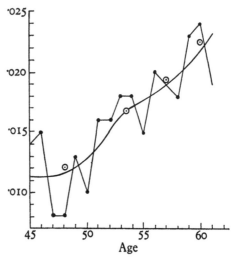

Fig. 7·1. Section of Sprague's graphic graduation of the mortality rates of the Government Annuitants' Experience, 1884, female lives, excluding the first 4 years after purchase.

7·14. Approximate confidence limits

It may sometimes be helpful in making a graphic graduation of a set of mortality rates to record on the graph at each age the points representing the limits corresponding to some standard of 'confidence interval' (or 'posterior probability interval'). There is usually no need for complete precision in computing these limits, and, provided that the actual deaths at any given age are not fewer than about 10, the confidence points, corresponding to an approximate 5 % confidence level, may be taken as $\mathring{q}_x \pm 2\sqrt{\theta_x/E_x}$. A jagged line can then be drawn through the set of upper limits and another such line through the set of lower limits. The jagged line representing $\mathring{q}_x$ would run between these two limit lines which would provide a convenient guide when drawing the smooth curve for the graduation. The smooth curve should not, of course, pass outside the limit points more often than about once in twenty ages, since the confidence level on which they are based is 5 %.

This procedure (which originated in principle with H. P. Calderon in *J.I.A.* **35**, 170, 1899) is really an alternative to Sprague's system of judiciously grouping the ages and then plotting the group-rates. The ranges of limits are not, of course, relevant to such group-points. Nor could any suitable confidence limits be computed for these group-rates because of the arbitrary balancing effect that would have been achieved in the selection of the ages for grouping. If, however, a uniform system of grouping were employed (e.g. quinary groups) a suitable set of approximate confidence limits would be given by

$$(\text{group } \mathring{q}) \pm 2\sqrt{(\text{group deaths})/(\text{group } E)}.$$

Whether the operator is helped by plotting the confidence limits is largely a matter of personal taste, but perhaps one advantage is that the confidence limits automatically provide a graphical expression of the weight of the data at the successive ages. In an unusual case where E_x shows large variations from age to age this might be of considerable importance in showing which observed rates should most influence the drawing of the smooth curve.

7·15. Tests of a graduation

As has already been mentioned, smoothness may be tested by taking out the successive differences of the graduated rates and seeing if they become small. Owing to the limitation in the number of significant figures used for the rates of mortality and the consequent rounding of the last recorded digit there is always a definite limit to the smoothness that can be expected in the differences. For example, it may be that the second or third differences are small and fluctuate in the last digit around zero. In such a case the subsequent differences may grow larger as a result of the building up of the rounding-off errors. This effect can be easily seen by differencing a table of 4-figure logarithms. In testing a graduation, therefore, we must be content if the second or third differences are small without showing any clearly defined waves. Sprague's graduation shows small second differences, but there are definite waves which a more drastic graduation would have removed. Their retention requires justification, and it is doubtful if the figures themselves provide such justification. Sprague himself appealed to the course of the rates in other experiences to justify certain wave features of his graduation, but some part of the roughness of his graduation is due to too little attention being paid to securing a proper junction between sections of the rates graduated separately on different scales. One of Sprague's dividing points was between ages 51 and 52 which explains the effects caused by the value of Δq_{51}.

In testing for 'goodness of fit' the natural starting point is to calculate what the deaths at each age would have been if the graduated rates had been exactly experienced and then to compare these numbers with the actual deaths. The product $E_x q_x$ is usually referred to as 'the expected deaths', but it is important to appreciate exactly what is meant by this phrase. It does *not* mean the deaths that would be expected if the graduated rates were the actual probabilities of death. Nor does it mean 'the most probable number of deaths'. The word 'expected' is used in the strict sense of mathematical expectation. That is, given that E_x lives are each independently subject to a probability of death* of q_x the probability of $0, 1, 2, \ldots, E_x$ deaths would follow the binomial law. The mean value or expectation of this probability distribution is $E_x q_x$, which is referred to as 'the expected deaths'. We are, therefore, led to consider the deviations of the actual deaths from the expected deaths and their probabilities of having occurred.

Let us consider first the total deaths $\Sigma \theta_x$. If the graduated rates q_x were strictly applicable we should not expect (in the ordinary sense) that $\Sigma \theta_x$ would exactly equal $\Sigma E_x q_x$, although this would be

---

* This statement is unnecessarily restrictive for the expected deaths for which all that is needed is that the average probability should be q_x, without even the conditions of independence. However, the conditions as stated are appropriate if the binomial is to be used for the variance.

the total expected deaths in the mean-value sense. Since the variance of the sum of a number of independent random variables is equal to the sum of the separate variances, the standard deviation of the total deaths would be $\sqrt{\Sigma(E_x p_x q_x)} \doteqdot \sqrt{\Sigma\theta_x}$. It would not be inappropriate, therefore, on a 1 in 20 approximate confidence level, for our graduated rates to be such that $\Sigma E_x q_x$ lay anywhere within the range $\Sigma\theta_x \pm 2\sqrt{\Sigma\theta_x}$. In practice, it is usual to avoid any bias one way or the other—although particular purposes may suggest that bias in one direction is very much to be preferred to bias in the other direction. Accordingly, in graduation work it is usual to endeavour to ensure that the total expected deaths closely approximate to the total actual deaths. Moreover, such a close approximation is desired for successive small age-ranges separately. The simplest way of testing for this is to calculate the individual deviations $\theta_x - E_x q_x = \delta_x$, and then to sum them continuously from the top or bottom of the table. It is then required of an acceptable graduation that δ_x should change sign frequently and that $\Sigma^x\delta_x$ should not build up to a large positive or negative figure at any age. It will usually be found that the accumulated deviations $\Sigma^x\delta_x$ do not change sign as frequently as δ_x, but several sign changes in a range of 50 ages would usually occur with a satisfactory graduation. Probability tests for the number of sign changes in δ_x and $\Sigma^x\delta_x$ have been devised, but they are ancillary to other tests which are usually sufficient in practical work.

Provided that each life appears only once in E_x, i.e. provided that there are no duplicates in the data, it is usually permissible to adopt the hypothesis that each deviation δ_x is a binomial variate which can be compared with the mean deviation $\cdot 8\sqrt{(E_x p_x q_x)}$, or with the standard deviation $\sqrt{(E_x p_x q_x)}$. On this basis only about 1 in 20 of the values of $|\delta_x|$ should be in excess of twice the corresponding standard deviation. An overall test can be made by comparing the total deviations irrespective of sign (i.e. $\Sigma|\delta_x|$) with the total of the mean deviations (i.e. $\cdot 8\Sigma\sqrt{(E_x p_x q_x)}$).

A more sophisticated test is the χ^2-test. On the binomial hypothesis the value of χ^2 at age x is $\delta_x^2/E_x p_x q_x$. The sum of the values of χ^2 for all ages, combining together any ages where the number of deaths is below, say, 8, may be compared with the expected χ^2-total, which is, of course, the number of individual values of χ^2. The question of constraints arises and there are two views. First, we may regard our actual data as a random sample from a universe subject to the rates of mortality q_x; on this view there are no constraints to be allowed for. The other view is that by making $\Sigma E_x q_x \doteqdot \Sigma \theta_x$ we have introduced one constraint, and that we should regard our set of deviations as a sample experiment from a set of possible experiments for each of which the graduated values are obtained subject to the condition $\Sigma E_x q_x = \Sigma \theta_x$. In practical work, the judgment of a graduation would not usually be influenced by such a relatively minute effect as a difference of one unit in the χ^2-total. Further information regarding the χ^2-test and the use of the corresponding probability tables is given in Johnson and Tetley's *Statistics* (Vol. II, Chaps. 11 and 12). The probability measures for the total mean deviation test together with a discussion and illustration of the relative results of these two tests and of a weighted χ^2-test and a standardized mean deviation test are given in R. E. Beard's paper entitled 'Some notes on graduation' (*J.I.A.* 77, 382).

7·16. Application of tests to the data in Table 7·3

The various tests may now be applied to the section of Sprague's graduation given in Table 7·3. The results are shown in Table 7·4. The deviations change sign nine times in sixteen ages. The accumulated deviations change sign six times and are never greater than about two individual deviations. The comparison of $\Sigma |\delta_x|$ with $\cdot 8 \Sigma \sqrt{(Epq)}$ shows a fair agreement and χ^2 at 17·8 compares well with 16 degrees of freedom. It may be noted here that not only should $\Sigma |\delta|$ and χ^2 not be too large but they should also not be too small. If the deviations as a whole were too small there would be strong evidence of undergraduation which would 'almost certainly' be evidenced also by lack of smoothness. If, however, the graduation survived the test of smoothness a small value of χ^2 would not, of itself, be a reason for rejecting the graduation. In the present case, the graduation survives the tests of goodness of fit but is lacking somewhat in smoothness. It is plain that improve-

TABLE 7·4. *Tests of 'goodness of fit' applied to the graduated rates given in Table 7·3*

Age x	Deviation δ_x	Accumulated deviation $\Sigma^x \delta_x$	$\sqrt{(E_x p_x q_x)}$	$\chi^2 = \delta_x^2 / E_x p_x q_x$
45	2·8	2·8	3·7	·6
46	5·0	7·8	4·0	1·6
47	−5·0	2·8	4·1	1·4
48	−6·3	−3·5	4·5	2·0
49	2·3	−1·2	4·8	·2
50	−6·1	−7·3	5·3	1·3
51	3·6	−3·7	5·7	·4
52	1·6	−2·1	6·4	·1
53	3·6	1·5	6·8	·3
54	2·4	3·9	7·5	·1
55	−8·2	−4·3	8·0	1·1
56	7·5	3·2	8·6	·7
57	·6	3·8	9·2	—
58	−7·2	−3·4	9·8	·5
59	13·2	9·8	10·3	1·6
60	14·4	24·2	11·0	1·7
61	−24·1	·1	11·7	4·2
	+57·0 −56·9		121·4	17·8

ment in the smoothness could be secured, either by hand-polishing the curve on the graph or by small adjustments to the graduated rates, and that this improvement could be achieved without any significant impairment of the fit.

7·17. Graduation by reference to a standard table

One of the simplest ways of graduating a set of mortality rates is to calculate at each age the value of $E_x q_x$, where q_x is the mortality rate according to some selected standard table. The ratio at each age of the actual deaths to the 'expected' deaths may then be graphed and a smooth curve drawn through the points representing the ratios. Graduated ratios would then be read off the graph and applied to the standard-table rates. The results would be the required graduated rates which would be tested in the usual way. Several trials and some hand-polishing might be necessary, and it would usually be helpful to combine the actual and expected deaths

H & P

in age-groups and obtain the corresponding group-ratios. These would then be represented on the graph as points corresponding to the mid-points of the age-groups. Obviously, the choice of a mortality table showing mortality rates not greatly different from the general level of the actual mortality rates to be graduated would be an advantage, and it is, of course, necessary that the standard table selected should be completely smooth.

7·18. General utility of graphic methods

Graphic methods of graduation are suitable for nearly all practical purposes. They may be applied to other mortality functions such as $\mathring{m}_x$, $\mathring{\mu}_x$, $\operatorname{colog}_e \mathring{p}_x$, $\log(\cdot 1 + \mathring{q}_x)$ and so on. The tests for 'goodness of fit' would in each case be made by reference to the actual and expected deaths. Graphic methods may also be applied to sickness, marriage and fertility rates, in fact to almost any kind of statistics where smoothing is required. If a very high degree of smoothness is required considerable hand-polishing may be necessary in the light of the run of the differences. In practice, it is difficult to read off a graph more than three significant figures, and if the degree of smoothness required suggests precision to a greater number of significant figures it may be necessary to resort to finite-difference methods, such as applying a low-powered summation formula to the rates as read off the graph. An alternative would be to read off graduated values at, say, every fifth age and then to apply the process of osculatory interpolation as described in the next chapter. Smoothness is a very desirable feature in a table that is to be used for the calculation of monetary functions, because anomalies in the run of the values may then be avoided and errors in calculations can be readily detected by differencing successive values of the tabulated functions. Smoothness is also a help if interpolation or quadrature formulae have to be applied to the table for particular purposes.

CHAPTER 8

PIVOTAL VALUES, OSCULATORY INTERPOLATION AND ABRIDGED LIFE TABLES

8·1. Pivotal values and osculatory interpolation

In §7·18 brief reference was made to the procedure of obtaining a set of graduated rates by reading values off a graph at intervals and then computing the intermediate values by osculatory interpolation. The 'pivotal values', as George King called them, may be obtained either by graphing the exposed-to-risk and deaths separately or by graphing the observed rates themselves. They may also be obtained in various other ways, and we shall now proceed to develop the finite-difference process which was used by George King for the English Life Tables Nos. 7 and 8 based on the 1911 census and which was subsequently used for the English Life Tables Nos. 9 and 10 based on the 1921 and 1931 censuses respectively. We shall then consider the process of osculatory interpolation.

8·2. Preliminary discussion

The origin of this pivotal-value process lay in the fact that the data of the earlier censuses were available only for age-groups, so that some distribution or interpolation process was essential. Then when the data were available in individual ages grouping in quinary groups was thought to be necessary to offset the systematic errors in the statement of age due to a preference by many people for particular final digits in the age such as 0, 5 and 8. Different quinary groupings were considered with the view to minimizing the extent of the overlap of errors from one age-group to the next.

In applying his process King followed precedent by operating separately on the numbers of populations and deaths, and at that time the assumption of a steady progression in the true numbers at successive ages was not, perhaps, unreasonable. For the 1921 tables a comparison was made between results based on the exposed-to-risk and deaths separately and the results obtained by operating on the rates directly. The differences proved to be of little significance. Owing to the considerable changes from year to year in the numbers of births during and since the 1914–18 war and the effect of the casualties in the two wars, it may be doubted whether a process dependent upon the assumption of a sufficient continuity in the run of the population totals over successive stretches of fifteen ages, which is the assumption underlying King's pivotal-value process, would nowadays be justified. Although the same methods were used in 1931 as in 1921 it seems possible that whatever methods may be used in future for the English Life Tables the graduation will be based on the rates directly.

Another consideration bearing on the methods used is the large number living at each age and the large number of deaths up to quite advanced ages. For a 3-year period the total number of deaths, males and females combined, in England and Wales is of the order of $1\frac{1}{2}$ millions. Apart, therefore, from the effect of age errors and of the irregularity in the numbers living at successive ages, the observed rates of mortality for quinary age-groups show a fairly regular progression even before graduation. For this reason and also because it is desired that the final tables should closely represent the actual mortality experienced, only a light graduation process is necessary, a process that does not iron out the wave-like features that are characteristic of the mortality experience of a large population such as that of Great Britain.

8·3. The pivotal-value formula

We now proceed to develop King's pivotal-value formula. For this purpose it is assumed that a given function u_{x+r} (that is to represent, for example, E_{x+r}, θ_{x+r} or $\mathring{q}_{x+r}$) is a third-degree function of r and that it is desired to obtain the value of u_{x+n} from grouped totals of u_{x+r} where the groups range over $2n+1$ values of r, e.g.

$W_0 = \sum_0^{2n} u_{x+r}$, $W_1 = \sum_{2n+1}^{4n+1} u_{x+r}$. If these grouped totals are continuously summed we may write

$$U_{-1} = \sum_{-(2n+1)}^{\omega} u_{x+r} = W_{-1} + W_0 + W_1 + \ldots,$$

$$U_0 = \sum_0^{\omega} u_{x+r} \qquad = W_0 + W_1 + W_2 + \ldots,$$

$$U_1 = \sum_{2n+1}^{\omega} u_{x+r} \quad = W_1 + W_2 + \ldots,$$

$$U_2 = \sum_{4n+2}^{\omega} u_{x+r} \quad = W_2 + \ldots,$$

where $x + \omega$ is the oldest age.

The pivotal-value formula required is a formula for the central value of u_{x+r} in each group-total, i.e. a formula for

$$u_{x+n} = (U_{n/(2n+1)} - U_{(n+1)/(2n+1)}).$$

Applying Bessel's interpolation formula (*Mathematics for Actuarial Students*, Part II, H. Freeman, p. 64) we have

$$U_{n/(2n+1)} = \tfrac{1}{2}(U_0 + U_1) + \left(\frac{n}{2n+1} - \frac{1}{2}\right)\Delta U_0$$

$$+ \frac{\left(\dfrac{n}{2n+1}\right)\left(\dfrac{n}{2n+1} - 1\right)}{2!} \frac{(\Delta^2 U_{-1} + \Delta^2 U_0)}{2}$$

$$+ \frac{\left(\dfrac{n}{2n+1} - \dfrac{1}{2}\right)\left(\dfrac{n}{2n+1}\right)\left(\dfrac{n}{2n+1} - 1\right)}{3!} \Delta^3 U_{-1} + \ldots,$$

$$U_{(n+1)/(2n+1)} = \tfrac{1}{2}(U_0 + U_1) + \left(\frac{n+1}{2n+1} - \frac{1}{2}\right)\Delta U_0$$

$$+ \frac{\left(\dfrac{n+1}{2n+1}\right)\left(\dfrac{n+1}{2n+1} - 1\right)}{2!} \frac{(\Delta^2 U_{-1} + \Delta^2 U_0)}{2}$$

$$+ \frac{\left(\dfrac{n+1}{2n+1} - \dfrac{1}{2}\right)\left(\dfrac{n+1}{2n+1}\right)\left(\dfrac{n+1}{2n+1} - 1\right)}{3!} \Delta^3 U_{-1} + \ldots.$$

Therefore

$$u_{x+n} = U_{n/(2n+1)} - U_{(n+1)/(2n+1)} = -\frac{1}{2n+1}\Delta U_0 + \frac{n(n+1)}{6(2n+1)^3}\Delta^3 U_{-1} \ldots.$$

A more general derivation of this formula is given in Johnson and Tetley's *Statistics*, Vol. I (p. 54). The formula may be written in a more familiar form by writing $m = 2n + 1$. We then have

$$u_{x + \frac{1}{2}(m-1)} = -\frac{1}{m}\left(\Delta U_0 - \frac{m^2 - 1}{24m^2}\Delta^3 U_{-1} + \ldots\right).$$

Putting $m = 5$ and writing W_0 for $-\Delta U_0$ and $\Delta^2 W_{-1}$ for $-\Delta^3 U_{-1}$, we reach King's pivotal-value formula for quinary groupings

$$u_{x+2} = \cdot 2W_0 - \cdot 008\Delta^2 W_{-1} + \ldots.$$

The pivotal-value formula could, of course, be applied to obtain a 'graduated' value of u_{x+r} for each value of r (apart from the first and last $m + n$ values of the whole set) by gradually moving up the age-groupings one age at a time. For example, with $m = 5$, q'_{27} could be obtained by grouping $\mathring{q}_x$ in the age-groups 20–24, 25–29, etc., while q'_{28} would require the age-groupings 21–25, 26–30, etc., and so on. In fact, as will be seen in Volume II the pivotal-value formula is a simple low-powered summation formula. The first term of the formula, i.e. W_0/m, is obviously a moving average extending over m terms. The second term of the formula is the adjustment necessary to offset the systematic second-difference error introduced by the moving average. In the example in §7.7 we applied a 5-year moving average to a series of values made up of a second-degree function plus an arbitrary error. The second-difference error $u'_x - u_x$ was equal to 1 at each age. In this example $\Delta^2 W_{-1} = 5^3 = 125$, and so if we had used King's formula instead of the simple moving average there would have been no systematic error introduced and each value of v'_x would have been 1 less. In practice, of course, we should not usually be working with a second-degree function plus an error, so that the results of applying King's formula would not be entirely free from systematic error. The formula is a central formula and is in fact correct to third differences. The remaining fourth-difference error is usually negligible for the type of data to which the formula is applied in practice. By extending Bessel's formula to include $\Delta^5 U_{-2}$ (i.e. to include the values of W_{-2} and W_2), King's formula can be made correct to fifth differences, but such meticulous accuracy would rarely be justified by the needs of the practical situation.

8·4. Osculatory interpolation

If pivotal values at intervals of m years of age have been obtained by graphical means or by King's formula or in some other way, it may be desired to interpolate values for each intermediate integral age. An ordinary interpolation formula could be used, but this would mean that the data used for the interpolation would gradually change as we passed to the higher ages. For example, we might have the pivotal values of q_x at ages 22, 27, 32, 37, etc. Then for q_{28}, q_{29}, q_{30} and q_{31} we might use a third-degree interpolation formula based on q_{22}, q_{27}, q_{32} and q_{37}. For the rates at ages 33–36 we should omit q_{22} and bring into account q_{42}, and for every succeeding gap to be filled we should omit one more pivotal value and bring in another. This process would tend to result in certain roughnesses in the first and second differences around the pivotal points as we change the data upon which the intermediate rates are based. In other words, the successive interpolation curves would intersect at the relevant pivotal ages, whereas for smoothness they should, of course, be tangential to each other. The extent of the disturbance obviously depends on the size of the third differences if these are the highest differences brought into account. To overcome this effect of simple interpolation special interpolation formulae have been devised which ensure continuity of the first derivatives of the overlapping interpolation curves. It is arranged for these curves to join smoothly or 'kiss'—hence the name 'osculatory interpolation'. Fifth-degree formulae have been devised to ensure continuity of the second as well as the first derivatives of the overlapping interpolation curves. It is rarely necessary to go to such lengths, and in fact in many cases the use of third-degree osculatory interpolation may be regarded as somewhat meticulous although it has been used for the English Life Tables 7 to 10.

One way, in fact the original way, of deriving an interpolation formula with osculatory properties is to make a suitable blend of two overlapping ordinary interpolation curves. Suppose that we wanted to interpolate values of u_x between u_0 and u_1 on the basis of given values of u_{-1}, u_0, u_1 and u_2. An ordinary third-degree interpolation formula would express the unique cubic that passes through these four values. To secure the osculatory property we have to waive some of the conditions upon which the ordinary interpolation curve depends and replace them by the desired osculatory conditions. What is done is to relax the condition that the interpolation curve must pass through u_{-1} and u_2. It is then possible to derive a cubic passing through u_0 and u_1 (but not through u_{-1} and u_2), which nevertheless is correct to *second* differences (i.e. it would reproduce u_{-1}, u_0, u_1 and u_2 if these were all points on a parabola), and which has the desired osculatory property (i.e. it has the same first derivative at $x=0$ as the corresponding interpolation curve for the interval -1 to 0 and similarly with regard to the first derivatives at 1).

We, therefore, start with the second-degree curve passing through u_{-1}, u_0 and u_1 and express this in the form of Gauss's 'backward' formula as follows:

$$(a) \quad u_x = u_0 + x\Delta u_{-1} + \frac{x(x+1)}{2}\Delta^2 u_{-1}.$$

Similarly, the second-degree curve passing through u_0, u_1 and u_2 may be expressed in the form of the advancing-difference formula as follows:

$$(b) \quad u_x = u_0 + x\Delta u_0 + \frac{x(x-1)}{2}\Delta^2 u_0$$

$$= u_0 + x\Delta u_{-1} + \frac{x(x+1)}{2}\Delta^2 u_{-1} + \frac{x(x-1)}{2}\Delta^3 u_{-1}.$$

The only difference between the two interpolation curves (a) and (b) is the third-difference term $x(x-1)\Delta^3 u_{-1}/2$ in (b). If u_{-1}, u_0, u_1 and u_2 were strictly parabolic $\Delta^3 u_{-1}$ would be zero, and the two interpolation curves would be identical and would pass through all four given values. In general, when the given values are not parabolic, any blend of the two interpolation curves would pass through u_0 and u_1 because the third-difference term in (b) vanishes for $x=0$ and $x=1$. A blend of the two interpolation curves would take the form $(1-p_x)\,(a) + p_x\,(b)$, where p_x would be some simple function of x. The required interpolation curve is therefore the second-difference formula (a) plus p_x times the third-difference term in (b). It will now be shown that the osculatory property at $x=0$ and $x=1$ applies if and only if $p_0=0$ and $p_1=1$.

The interpolation curve for the interval o to 1 is

$$u_x = u_0 + x\Delta u_{-1} + \frac{x(x+1)}{2}\Delta^2 u_{-1} + \frac{x(x-1)}{2}p_x\Delta^3 u_{-1},$$

so that

$$\frac{du_x}{dx} = \Delta u_{-1} + \frac{2x+1}{2}\Delta^2 u_{-1} + \frac{2x-1}{2}p_x\Delta^3 u_{-1} + \frac{dp_x}{dx}\frac{x(x-1)}{2}\Delta^3 u_{-1}.$$

We, therefore, have

$$\left[\frac{du_x}{dx}\right]_{x=0} = \Delta u_{-1} + \tfrac{1}{2}\Delta^2 u_{-1} - \tfrac{1}{2}p_0\Delta^3 u_{-1}, \tag{A}$$

$$\left[\frac{du_x}{dx}\right]_{x=1} = \Delta u_{-1} + \tfrac{3}{2}\Delta^2 u_{-1} + \tfrac{1}{2}p_1\Delta^3 u_{-1}, \tag{B}$$

provided that p_0' and p_1' do not diverge. Similarly, for the interpolation curve for the interval -1 to o we have

$$\left[\frac{du_{-1+x}}{dx}\right]_{x=1} = \Delta u_{-2} + \tfrac{3}{2}\Delta^2 u_{-2} + \tfrac{1}{2}p_1\Delta u_{-2}, \tag{C}$$

and for the interpolation curve for the interval 1 to 2 we have

$$\left[\frac{du_{1+x}}{dx}\right]_{x=0} = \Delta u_0 + \tfrac{1}{2}\Delta^2 u_0 - \tfrac{1}{2}p_0\Delta^3 u_0. \tag{D}$$

The osculatory conditions may be expressed as

$$A = C \quad \text{and} \quad B = D,$$

i.e. $\quad \Delta u_{-1} + \tfrac{1}{2}\Delta^2 u_{-1} - \tfrac{1}{2}p_0\Delta^3 u_{-1} = \Delta u_{-2} + \tfrac{3}{2}\Delta^2 u_{-2} + \tfrac{1}{2}p_1\Delta^3 u_{-2}$

and $\quad \Delta u_{-1} + \tfrac{3}{2}\Delta^2 u_{-1} + \tfrac{1}{2}p_1\Delta^3 u_{-1} = \Delta u_0 + \tfrac{1}{2}\Delta^2 u_0 - \tfrac{1}{2}p_0\Delta^3 u_0.$

From the first of these two equations we have

$$\Delta^3 u_{-2} = p_0\Delta^3 u_{-1} + p_1\Delta^3 u_{-2},$$

and from the second we have

$$\Delta^3 u_{-1} = p_0\Delta^3 u_0 + p_1\Delta^3 u_{-1}.$$

Hence $\qquad\qquad p_0 = 0 \quad \text{and} \quad p_1 = 1.$

For reasons of symmetry, it seems appropriate that the interpolated value of $u_{\frac{1}{2}}$ should be $\tfrac{1}{2}(a) + \tfrac{1}{2}(b)$ so that $p_{\frac{1}{2}}$ would be ·5. The simplest form for p_x which fulfils the required conditions is

$p_x = x$. This form is also the only possible form for p_x if we stipulate that the interpolation curve must be a cubic. The symmetrical third-degree osculatory interpolation formula correct to second differences for the interval o to 1 is therefore

$$u_x = u_0 + x\Delta u_{-1} + \frac{x(x+1)}{2}\Delta^2 u_{-1} + \frac{x^2(x-1)}{2}\Delta^3 u_{-1},$$

which is in the form given by Lidstone in *J.I.A.* **42**, 394.

Any other blending function such that $p_0 = 0$, $p_{\frac{1}{2}} = \cdot 5$ and $p_1 = 1$ could be used, but the resulting formula would not then be of the third degree. It can easily be shown that if we choose a blending function such that its derivatives at o and 1 vanish, then the resulting interpolation formula has the further property of second-order contact, i.e. the second derivatives at o and 1 are equal to the second derivatives of the corresponding interpolation curves for the adjacent intervals. A blending function with this further property is $p_x = 3x^2 - 2x^3$. The 'curve of sines' used in connexion with the English Life Table No. 5 (see § 9·1) also provides first- and second-order contact. However, if third-degree interpolation is adequate for a particular purpose, it may be doubted whether the improvement in results achieved by these refinements would be worth the trouble involved. Usually, if better results are required an interpolation formula of a higher degree must be used. T. B. Sprague originally devised his fifth-degree formula on the basis of given values of u_0, u_1, u'_0, u''_0, u'_1 and u''_1. These first and second derivatives were based on the respective fourth-degree curves passing through u_{-2}, u_{-1}, u_0, u_1 and u_2 and u_{-1}, u_0, u_1, u_2 and u_3. It was subsequently shown that the resulting osculatory interpolation formula was in fact correct to fourth differences. This is the way in which osculatory interpolation formulae have usually been derived, and it is the way used by King for the third-degree formula employed in the construction of the English Life Tables Nos. 7–10. It is also the way used by H. Freeman in *Mathematics for Actuarial Students*, Vol. II, p. 147. H. Vaughan has recently pointed out (*J.I.A.* **80**, 63) that this method of derivation does not bring out the uniqueness of each formula in the prescribed conditions nor the necessity of the formula being correct to second or fourth differences, as the case may be. This criticism is perfectly valid, and Vaughan's note—to which we are indebted—throws a good deal of fresh light on the whole subject of osculatory interpolation. Nevertheless, the traditional approach has the merit that it shows that the values of the derivatives imposed upon the interpolation curve at $x=0$ and $x=1$ are, in fact, suitable values. Accordingly, we include a brief derivation of King's formula (in Lidstone's form) on the traditional lines.

We again assume that u_{-1}, u_0, u_1 and u_2 are given, that interpolated values between $x=0$ and $x=1$ are required, and that the interpolation curve is to pass through u_0 and u_1 but not necessarily through u_{-1} and u_2.

u_0' is to be based on u_{-1}, u_0 and u_1, i.e.

$$\left[\frac{du_x}{dx}\right]_{x=0} = \left[\frac{d}{dx}\left(u_0 + x\Delta u_{-1} + \frac{x(x+1)}{2}\Delta^2 u_{-1}\right)\right]_{x=0}$$
$$= [\Delta u_{-1} + (x+\tfrac{1}{2})\Delta^2 u_{-1}]_{x=0}$$
$$= \Delta u_{-1} + \tfrac{1}{2}\Delta^2 u_{-1}$$
$$= \tfrac{1}{2}(u_1 - u_{-1}).$$

u_1' is to be based on u_0, u_1 and u_2, i.e.

$$\left[\frac{du_x}{dx}\right]_{x=1} = \Delta u_0 + \tfrac{1}{2}\Delta^2 u_0$$
$$= \tfrac{1}{2}(u_2 - u_0).$$

The required third-degree interpolation formula may be written in the form $\qquad u_x = a + bx + cx^2 + dx^3,$

and the four conditions give the following equations

$$u_0 = a,$$
$$u_1 = a + b + c + d,$$
$$u_0' = \Delta u_{-1} + \tfrac{1}{2}\Delta^2 u_{-1} = b,$$
$$u_1' = \Delta u_0 + \tfrac{1}{2}\Delta^2 u_0 = b + 2c + 3d.$$

Hence $c = \tfrac{1}{2}(\Delta^2 u_{-1} - \Delta^3 u_{-1})$ and $d = \tfrac{1}{2}\Delta^3 u_{-1}$, and we reach the same third-degree formula as before, i.e.

$$u_x = u_0 + x\Delta u_{-1} + \frac{x(x+1)}{2}\Delta^2 u_{-1} + \frac{x^2(x-1)}{2}\Delta^3 u_{-1}.$$

It is interesting to compare the osculatory formula with the corresponding ordinary interpolation formula for which the third-difference term is $\dfrac{x(x^2-1)}{6}\Delta^3 u_{-1}$. The difference between the two is therefore $\dfrac{x(x-1)(2x-1)}{6}\Delta^3 u_{-1}$, which shows the third-difference error introduced to secure osculation. It is of interest to compare this error with the coefficient of the third difference as shown in Table 8·1.

TABLE 8·1

x	$\dfrac{x(x^2-1)}{6}$	$\dfrac{x(x-1)(2x-1)}{6}$	x	$\dfrac{x(x^2-1)}{6}$	$\dfrac{x(x-1)(2x-1)}{6}$
·1	−·0165	·012	·6	−·0640	−·008
·2	−·0320	·016	·7	−·0595	−·014
·3	−·0455	·014	·8	−·0480	−·016
·4	−·0560	·008	·9	−·0285	−·012
·5	−·0625	—			

It may be argued that just as the error introduced by an osculatory formula is small, so also, up to a point, must be the improvement in the smoothness. We must bear in mind, however, that an improvement in smoothness may significantly affect the third differences while only slightly affecting the rates themselves. We may obtain a general idea of the magnitude of the osculatory adjustment for mortality rates by considering an example in which we are given quinary pivotal values of μ_x which follow Makeham's law. If $\mu_x = A + Bc^x$

$$\Delta^3 \mu_{x-5} \doteq h^3 \mu'''_{x+2\frac{1}{2}} = 125 Bc^{x+2\frac{1}{2}} \log_e^3 c.$$

The range of the osculatory adjustment is therefore

$$\pm \cdot 016 \times 125 \times Bc^{x+2\frac{1}{2}} \log_e^3 c$$
$$= \pm 2 \log_e^3 c\,(\mu_{x+2\frac{1}{2}} - A)$$
$$\doteq \pm \cdot 002\,(\mu_{x+2\frac{1}{2}} - A),$$

since $\log_e c$ is usually in the neighbourhood of ·1.

The conclusion to be drawn is that neither the error introduced by an osculatory formula nor the improvement in smoothness is of any great significance having regard to the roughnesses in the pivotal values obtained by using King's formula and to the resulting waves in the interpolated rates of mortality. Various refinements of the technique of osculatory interpolation have been devised, including higher-powered formulae that do not exactly reproduce any of the pivotal values and accordingly have a certain graduating effect. Particulars of their development are given by Freeman (loc. cit.).

8·5. Abridged life tables

It may sometimes be desired to use a set of pivotal values of q_x to provide values of l_x and e_x of the corresponding life table at every fifth age. In fact, given l_x at quinary intervals it is possible, by the use of quadrature and other finite-difference formulae, to approximate fairly closely to the various functions of the life table including monetary functions. George King devised a method of passing directly from quinary pivotal values of q_x to an abridged life table without going through the tedious process of interpolating individual values of q_x.

Since $l_{x+5} = {}_5p_x l_x$, the problem of constructing an abridged life table, starting with a suitable radix l_α at the initial age α, is essentially the problem of computing the values of ${}_5p_x$ at quinary intervals of x. The function ${}_5p_x$ is the product $p_x p_{x+1} \dots p_{x+4}$, and so by taking logarithms we have

$$\log {}_5p_x = \sum_r^4 \log p_{x+r} = \sum_r^4 \log (1 - q_{x+r}).$$

Writing u_{x+r} for $\log p_{x+r}$, the problem is to find a formula for $\sum_r^4 u_{x+r}$ in terms of quinary values of u_{x+r}. It is convenient to use 5 years as the unit of measurement, and we assume that u_r is given for $r = -1$, o, 1 and 2 and that we desire to approximate to

$$u_0 + u_{.2} + u_{.4} + u_{.6} + u_{.8}.$$

Then by using the advancing-difference formula

$$u_r \doteqdot u_{-1} + (r+1)\Delta u_{-1} + \frac{(r+1)r}{2!}\Delta^2 u_{-1} + \frac{(r+1)r(r-1)}{3!}\Delta^3 u_{-1},$$

we obtain King's formula

$$u_0 + u_{.2} + u_{.4} + u_{.6} + u_{.8} \doteqdot 5u_{-1} + 7\Delta u_{-1} + 1\cdot 6\Delta^2 u_{-1} - \cdot 2\Delta^3 u_{-1}$$
$$= -\cdot 2u_{-1} + 3\cdot 2u_0 + 2\cdot 2u_1 - \cdot 2u_2.$$

This formula enables us to obtain a value for $_5p_x$ from q_{x-5}, q_x, q_{x+5} and q_{x+10}, but it does not provide the value of $_5p_{x-5}$ for the initial quinary interval. Using the same advancing-difference formula the required formula is

$$u_{-1\cdot0} + u_{-\cdot8} + u_{-\cdot6} + u_{-\cdot4} + u_{-\cdot2} \doteq 5u_{-1} + 2\Delta u_{-1} - \cdot4\Delta^2 u_{-1} + \cdot2\Delta^3 u_{-1}$$

$$= 2\cdot4u_{-1} + 3\cdot4u_0 - 1\cdot0u_1 + \cdot2u_2.$$

In connexion with the construction of a service table for use in pension-fund work, H. Freeman (*J.I.A.* **61**, 9) suggested a simple process that can be adapted to the purpose of constructing an abridged life table. It is not, of course, as accurate as King's third-degree formulae, but it may often provide results that are accurate enough in practice. The principle of the method is to assume that $p_{x+1}p_{x+4} \doteq p_x p_{x+5}$ (i.e. one age down and one up) and that $p_{x+2}p_{x+3} \doteq p_x p_{x+5}$ (i.e. two ages down and two up). Then

$$\sum_0^4 \log p_{x+r} \doteq 3 \log p_x + 2 \log p_{x+5}$$

$$= 3u_0 + 2u_1$$

$$= 5u_{-1} + 7\Delta u_{-1} + 2\Delta^2 u_{-1} + 0.\Delta^3 u_{-1}.$$

Freeman's formula can be used for the initial interval. Expressing it in a form comparable with King's formula for the initial interval we have

$$3u_{-1} + 2u_0 = 5u_{-1} + 2\Delta u_{-1} + 0.\Delta^2 u_{-1} + 0.\Delta^3 u_{-1}.$$

King's formula is, of course, not quite central and, if the quinary age-points of the abridged table can be freely selected, it might be better to increase them by half a year and thereby make the table intervals central to the pivotal values. King's formula may then be adapted to produce $\log_5 p_{x+\frac{1}{2}}$, and the resulting formula is

$$u_{\cdot1} + u_{\cdot3} + u_{\cdot5} + u_{\cdot7} + u_{\cdot9} \doteq 5u_{-1} + 7\cdot5\Delta u_{-1} + 2\cdot075\Delta^2 u_{-1} - \cdot2125\Delta^3 u_{-1}$$

$$= -\cdot2125u_{-1} + 2\cdot7125u_0 + 2\cdot7125u_1 - \cdot2125u_2.$$

Freeman's formula for $\log_5 p_{x+\frac{1}{2}}$ would be

$$2\tfrac{1}{2}u_0 + 2\tfrac{1}{2}u_1 = 5u_{-1} + 7\cdot5\Delta u_{-1} + 2\cdot5\Delta^2 u_{-1} + 0.\Delta^3 u_{-1}.$$

Another approach would be to select the quinary age-intervals for the abridged table so that the intervals to which the pivotal values of q_x relate are central to the individual quinary intervals, that is, to approximate to $\log {}_5p_{x-2}$. This would be a very convenient arrangement if the quinary values had been obtained from the age-groupings 20–24, 25–29, etc., thus producing values of q_{22}, q_{27}, etc. The abridged table would then show values of l_{20}, l_{25}, etc. On this basis we can write down a formula of the type of Freeman's formula, viz.

$$\log {}_5p_{x-2} \doteqdot 5 \log p_x = 5u_0 = 5u_{-1} + 5\Delta u_{-1}.$$

The corresponding King-type formula would be

$$u_{-.4} + u_{-.2} + u_0 + u_{.2} + u_{.4} \doteqdot 5u_{-1} + 5\Delta u_{-1} + \cdot 2\Delta^2 u_{-1} + 0 . \Delta^3 u_{.1}$$
$$= \tfrac{1}{5}(u_{-1} + 23u_0 + u_1).$$

It may be useful to record the general formula of which this is a special case. It is to express $\sum_{-n}^{n} u_r$ in terms of the three values $u_{-(2n+1)}$, u_0 and u_{2n+1}. Using Taylor's theorem we have

$$u_r = u_0 + rD + \frac{r^2}{2!}D^2 + \frac{r^3 D^3}{3!} + \dots,$$

where $D^s = \left[\dfrac{d^s u_r}{dr^s}\right]_{r=0}$, so that

$$\sum_{-n}^{n} u_r = (2n+1)u_0 + \frac{n(n+1)(2n+1)}{6}D^2 + \dots.$$

To third differences

$$D^2 \doteqdot (u_{2n+1} - 2u_0 + u_{-(2n+1)})/(2n+1)^2$$

so that

$$\sum_{-n}^{n} u_r \doteqdot (2n+1)u_0 + \frac{n(n+1)}{6(2n+1)}(u_{2n+1} - 2u_0 + u_{-(2n+1)}).$$

8·6. The use of Makeham's formula in the construction of an abridged table

Instead of using ordinary finite-difference methods an abridged life table could be constructed by assuming that successive stretches of the table follow Makeham's formula. Thus if we are given q_{x-5}, q_x and q_{x+5} we can use these values to solve for the Makeham constants and then compute $_5p_x$. Taking x as the origin so that $l_{x+r} = ks^r g^{c^r}$, let

$$u_{-1} = \text{colog}_e p_{x-5} = -\log_e s - c^{-5}(c-1)\log_e g,$$
$$u_0 = \text{colog}_e p_x = -\log_e s - (c-1)\log_e g,$$
$$u_1 = \text{colog}_e p_{x+5} = -\log_e s - c^5(c-1)\log_e g.$$

Then
$$c^5 = \frac{\Delta u_0}{\Delta u_{-1}}, \quad \log_e g = -\frac{\Delta u_{-1}\Delta u_0}{(c-1)(\Delta^2 u_{-1})}$$

and
$$\log_e s = \frac{\Delta u_{-1}\Delta u_0}{\Delta^2 u_{-1}} - u_0.$$

Hence
$$\log_e {}_5p_x = \frac{5\Delta u_{-1}\Delta u_0}{\Delta^2 u_{-1}} - 5u_0 - \frac{\Delta u_0}{c-1}.$$

The same process can be used to obtain $_5p_{x+5}$, $_5p_{x+10}$ and so on.

8·7. Computation of $\bar{e}_x$ and $\bar{a}_x$ from an abridged table

As indicated in § 8·5 it is possible to approximate to various life-table functions on the basis of quinary values of l_{x+r}. Various quadrature formulae can be used, but we will illustrate by giving two processes of obtaining quinary values of $\bar{e}_x$ and $\bar{a}_x$ which are often the main objective of constructing an abridged table. The first process is to utilize the usual approximations to $\bar{e}_x$ and $\bar{a}_x$ but taking 5 years as the time unit—these approximations are, of course, based on the Euler-Maclaurin expansion. We then have

$$\bar{e}_x \doteq 5[(l_{x+5} + l_{x+10} + \ldots)/l_x + \tfrac{1}{2} - \tfrac{5}{12}\mu_x]$$

and
$$\bar{a}_x \doteq 5\,[(D_{x+5} + D_{x+10} + \ldots)/D_x + \tfrac{1}{2} - \tfrac{5}{12}(\mu_x + \delta)].$$

When summing l_x and D_x at yearly intervals the term in μ_x can usually be omitted, but with quinary intervals the term is more important. At most ages, however, it would be sufficient to substitute q_x for μ_x. If values of μ are required we can approximate by interpolating between successive quinary values of $\text{colog}_e p_x \doteq \mu_{x+\frac{1}{2}}$.

The alternative approach is to approximate to e_x by applying King's formula to obtain

$$T_{x\,\overline{5}|} = \sum_0^4 l_{x+r}, \quad T_{x+5\,\overline{5}|} = \sum_5^9 l_{x+r} \quad \text{and so on.}$$

Then
$$1 + e_x = (T_{x\,\overline{5}|} + T_{x+5\,\overline{5}|} + T_{x+10\,\overline{5}|} + \ldots)/l_x.$$

Similarly, for $(1 + a_x)$ we can use King's formula to approximate to $N_{x\,\overline{5}|} = \sum_0^4 D_{x+r}$ and so on.

CHAPTER 9

THE ENGLISH LIFE TABLES

9·1. The early English Life Tables

The series of life tables known as the English Life Tables have
been constructed on the basis of the census and deaths records over
the last 100 years as compiled and published by the General
Register Office. The first pair of tables, for males and females
separately, were constructed by Dr William Farr by relating the
numbers of deaths in the single year 1841 to the census figures for
the same year. This pair of tables are known as the English Life
Tables No. 1. Subsequently, Dr Farr used the same census
figures as the basis for the E.L.T. No. 2 in conjunction with the
average of the numbers of deaths for the 7-year period 1838–44,
of which the middle year was the census year. Later still, he used
the 1841 census yet again in constructing E.L.T. No. 3. For these
tables he related the numbers of deaths for the 17-year period
1838–54 to the mean populations, for the period covered by the
deaths, estimated for the relevant age-groups on the basis of the
census figures for 1841 and for 1851.

The principles used by Dr Farr were essentially the same as those
used for all subsequent tables, although there have, of course, been
various improvements of technique for the later tables. These
principles comprise the determination of mortality rates at pivotal
ages from the census and deaths figures grouped in age-groups, the
interpolation of the mortality rates for the intermediate ages, the
extension of the table at the oldest ages by some simple extrapolation process and the completion of the table at the youngest ages by
reference to the records of births and deaths in the relevant periods.

Following Farr's E.L.T. No. 3 no further national life tables
were constructed until after the 1881 census when the E.L.T. No. 4
were constructed on the basis of the censuses for the two years 1871
and 1881 and the numbers of deaths for the decennium 1871–80.
Then followed E.L.T. No. 5, based on the censuses of 1881 and

1891 and the deaths for 1881–1890. But none of these tables took the place of E.L.T. No. 3 (males) which had been fairly extensively used for certain actuarial purposes, notably in connexion with industrial life assurance. The male table for the next decennium, E.L.T. No. 6, based on the 1891 and 1901 censuses and the deaths for the decennium 1891–1900, was, however, more extensively used for actuarial purposes and largely replaced E.L.T. No. 3 in industrial assurance work. A combined table for males and females was also constructed and this table, known as E.L.T. No. 6 (persons), is enshrined in the Industrial Assurance Act, 1923 as the mortality basis for the statutory minimum free policy and surrender values prescribed in that Act for industrial assurance policies.

The technical details of the construction of these early tables is of little interest today, and we shall confine ourselves to mentioning that for E.L.T. No. 5 a process of blending overlapping interpolation curves was devised which, as we have seen, is a simple way of looking at the process of osculatory interpolation. The blending curve used for E.L.T. No. 5 was based on the curve of sines, the range of the blending being ten ages and the proportions of the two interpolated values being taken as $\frac{1}{2}(1 \pm \cos\frac{1}{10}t\pi)$ $(0 \leqslant t \leqslant 10)$. This blend line has the same properties as the blend line $3x^2 - 2x^3$ $(0 \leqslant x \leqslant 1)$ mentioned in §8·4, namely, $p_0 = 0$, $p_{10} = 1$, $p_5 = \frac{1}{2}$ and $p_0' = p_{10}' = 0$.

9·2. English Life Tables Nos. 7 and 8

The process of obtaining pivotal values by finite-difference methods from the national census and deaths records and the process of completing the table by osculatory interpolation were considered in detail by George King in a series of papers read before the Institute of Actuaries in which he also discussed the methods used for the earlier tables. Osculatory interpolation had been earlier developed by T. B. Sprague. When the 1911 census results became available George King was accordingly entrusted with the task of constructing new national life tables for which he proceeded to use his own methods (*Supplement to the Seventy-fifth Annual Report of the Registrar-General*, Part I, Life Tables). With minor modifications these methods have since been used for subsequent tables

(E.L.T. Nos. 9 and 10), and they have also been used for life tables for various sections of the population and in certain other countries as well.

King constructed two sets of tables—E.L.T. No. 7 based on the two censuses of 1901 and 1911 and the deaths for the years 1901–10, and E.L.T. No. 8 based on the single census of 1911 and the deaths for the three years 1910–12.

For E.L.T. No. 7 the possible procedures were conditioned by the fact that the 1901 census figures were tabulated in the last birthday age-groups 5–9, 10–14, ..., 95–99 with a final group for ages 100 and over. King accordingly grouped the 1911 census figures in the same age-groups and then obtained from the group figures for the two censuses mean populations as estimates of one-tenth of the central exposed-to-risk for each age-group for the decennium covered by the deaths. The principles used in obtaining the mean populations had been devised by A. C. Waters of the General Register Office and had been used for E.L.T. No. 5. The assumptions made were: (1) that the total population increased in geometrical progression from the first census to the second census and (2) that the proportion of persons in a given age-group to the total changed in arithmetical progression from the first census to the second census. The assumed annual rate of progression of the total population was easily obtained from $r^{10} = \sum_x P_x(1911)/\sum_x P_x(1901)$. Writing α_0 and α_{10} for the proportions of the total populations at 1901 and 1911 respectively for a given age-group and T for the total population at 1901, the estimate of the population in the age-group at time t was then given by $\quad [\alpha_0 + \cdot 1 t(\alpha_{10} - \alpha_0)](Tr^t),$

and the central exposed-to-risk for the age-group for the decennium was given by the integral

$$\int_0^{10} [\alpha_0 + \cdot 1 t(\alpha_{10} - \alpha_0)] Tr^t dt$$

$$= \frac{\alpha_0 T(r^{10} - 1)}{\log_e r} + \frac{(\alpha_{10} - \alpha_0) T}{\log_e r} \left[r^{10} - \frac{r^{10} - 1}{10 \log_e r} \right]$$

$$= \lambda^{-1} [\cdot 1 \lambda^{-1}(r^{10} - 1) - 1] \cdot {}_0 P + \lambda^{-1} [1 - \cdot 1 \lambda^{-1}(1 - r^{-10})] \cdot {}_{10} P$$

$$= k \cdot {}_0 P + l \cdot {}_{10} P,$$

where $\lambda = \log_e r$, $_0P$ is the population in the given age-group at the first census, $_{10}P$ is the population in the given age-group at the second census and k and l are independent of age and are functions only of r, i.e. of the total populations. As the 1901 and 1911 censuses were taken on 31 March and 2 April respectively the exposed-to-risk figures were actually obtained by taking $-\frac{1}{4}$ and $9\frac{3}{4}$ as the limits of the integrals instead of 0 and 10.

It may be doubted whether all this trouble was worth while or whether in fact the process did not involve a significant element of spurious accuracy, particularly when we bear in mind the rapid growth of the population over the period, the somewhat irregular course of the numbers in a given age-group as the years go by, the considerable age-errors that existed in the census figures and the considerable fluctuations and seasonal variations that occurred in the numbers of deaths. Be that as it may, the No. 7 tables have never been used very much except to provide additional sets of rates when considering the trend of mortality over the years.

Apart from the doubts about the suitability of basing a table on the deaths for such a long period as 10 years and the figures of two censuses 10 years apart, such a table is already well over 5 years out of date by the time that it can be constructed. For these and other reasons George King decided to construct E.L.T. No. 8 based on the deaths for the 3 years 1910–12, and the single census of 1911. The question at once arises of whether 3 years provides a sufficient balance between good and bad mortality years to permit the resulting table to be reasonably representative of the period. This question is the more important because a 3-year period was subsequently used both for E.L.T. No. 9 and for E.L.T. No. 10. The answer depends upon the general level of the mortality of the years concerned when considered in relation to the surrounding years. From this point of view the three periods 1910–12, 1920–22, 1930–32 were probably reasonably representative, although it should be noted that not only were the influenza epidemics of 1918/19 and 1929 totally excluded, but the years immediately following the epidemics, which were particularly light mortality years, were included.

The 1911 census figures were adjusted to allow for the period from the census date 2 April to 30 June 1911 which was the mid-point of the 3-year period to which the deaths for E.L.T. No. 8 were to relate. The adjustment was based on the common ratio r computed for E.L.T. No. 7. The central exposed-to-risk were then taken as three times the adjusted census figures. As these figures were available for each age it was possible to choose any form of grouping of the ages. George King considered the incidence of the age-errors and the best way to combine the ages so as to offset these errors. He finally chose the groupings 4–8, 9–13, etc. This is a sensible arrangement if there is reason to suppose that there is a tendency to favour ages ending in 0 and 5 and to a less extent 2 and 8.

There are other kinds of age-errors which no amount of grouping will offset because they are biased in one direction. These errors include the tendency for women, particularly in middle age, to understate their ages deliberately even in census returns, and the tendency for elderly people to exaggerate their ages. The extent and incidence of these various errors in the census and deaths returns were considered in 1927 by V. P. A. Derrick in a paper submitted to the Institute of Actuaries (*J.I.A.* **58**, 117). National Insurance, the National Registration of 1939, rationing, special benefits for old people and so on—all these, together with a more educated approach to such matters as censuses and death registrations, have no doubt contributed to reduce the significance of these age-errors in more recent years to such an extent that the Registrar-General's estimated population figures for inter-censal years, computed by reference to the birth, death and migration records, have shown a fairly close agreement with the subsequent census figures of 1951. It may be, therefore, that age-errors will play a less significant part in determining the details of construction of future national life tables. On the other hand, the irregularities in the age-progression of the census figures, due to such features as changes in the numbers of births from year to year and war casualties, suggest that methods dependent upon an assumption of an underlying regularity of the numbers at successive ages may need reconsideration.

9·3. English Life Tables Nos. 9 and 10

These tables were constructed by the Government Actuary, Sir Alfred Watson, by the same methods as were used by King for E.L.T. No. 8. The No. 9 tables (*The Registrar-General's Decennial Supplement*, 1921, Part I, Life Tables) were based on the 1921 census and the numbers of deaths in the years 1920–22. The No. 10 tables (*The Registrar-General's Decennial Supplement* 1931, Part I, Life Tables) were based on the 1931 census and the numbers of deaths in the years 1930–32. On each occasion Watson re-examined the question of the most suitable age-grouping for counteracting age-errors. For the 1921 census figures and for the deaths for the years 1920–22 the Registrar-General had already considered this question and had suggested that the irregularities in the numbers of deaths and in the census figures generally corresponded with each other. After experiment, therefore, Watson adopted the grouping that the Registrar-General had suggested, namely, 2–6, 7–11, 12–16 and so on. For E.L.T. No. 10 the grouping adopted, on a balance of considerations, was 5–9, 10–14 and so on.

The 1921 census was taken on the night of 19–20 June, and as this was only 11 days from the mid-point of the year the central exposed-to-risk for the period 1920–22 were taken as three times the unadjusted census figures. The 1931 census was taken on the night of 26–27 April. Although this was 65 days before the mid-point of the year, the unadjusted census figures were again taken as the basis of the mean populations. Watson pointed out that the progression of the population from 1921 to 1931 varied considerably from age-group to age-group and gave no reliable measure of the progression in the early part of the next decennium, and he drew attention to the irregularities in the numbers at successive ages. He concluded that there was no basis for making a reliable adjustment of the census figures to the mid-point of the year, that in any case the population figures at the mid-point of the year, if known, would provide only approximations to the mean populations for the 3-year period of the deaths, and that any suitable adjustments would have only trifling effects on the resulting rates of mortality.

Both for E.L.T. No. 9 and for E.L.T. No. 10 pivotal values were obtained separately for the mean populations and for the numbers of deaths. The pivotal rates of mortality at the quinary age-points were obtained by division, and the rates for the intermediate ages were obtained by using King's third-degree osculatory-inter-polation formula.

As an experiment in connexion with E.L.T. No. 9 Watson computed the ungraduated rates of mortality at each age, combined these in quinary age-groups and applied King's pivotal formula to produce alternative pivotal mortality rates. He compared these rates with the corresponding graduated rates obtained by operating on the census and deaths figures separately. The differences were small and unimportant. He did not repeat the experiment for E.L.T. No. 10 for which pivotal values of the census and deaths figures were again separately computed.

In view of the irregularity of the numbers in the population at successive ages and, hence, of the corresponding deaths figures, the validity of the application of the assumptions underlying King's finite-difference pivotal-value formula may be seriously questioned. No doubt the ratio of the number of deaths in a 5-year age-group to the mean population in the same 5-year age-group provides a reasonably valid estimate of $\mathring{m}_x$ for some age-point close to the mid-point of the age-range, dependent upon the way in which the lives are distributed over the individual ages in the group. It is the fact that the second-difference term in King's formula is obtained from the set of irregular numbers that provides the reason for doubt. And yet it may be that by applying this second-difference adjustment both to the numbers of deaths and to the census figures there may be some compensation for the disturbing effects of the irregularities. Watson mentioned in connexion with E.L.T. No. 10 that the irregularities in the deaths and census figures generally correspond to each other, and it would seem, therefore, that a more valid process might be to follow the lines of the experiment made in connexion with E.L.T. No. 9 and operate on the mortality rates for the individual ages instead of on the census and deaths figures separately. It might in fact be better to adapt an idea used by Watson in connexion with the computation of the rates for ages 6–16 (see § 9·5) for E.L.T. No. 10

by substituting $(P_{x-1}+P_x+P_{x+1})$ for $3P_x$ as the estimate of the exposed-to-risk at age x in obtaining $\mathring{m}_x$. In this way allowance would be made for the disturbances due to fluctuations in births and war casualties. The reason for this may be seen in the following way. If censuses were taken on 1 July of each year the exposed-to-risk corresponding to the deaths at age x in the 3-year period would naturally be taken as $(\frac{1}{2}P_x+1\frac{1}{2}P_x+2\frac{1}{2}P_x)$. By using $(1\frac{1}{2}P_{x-1}+1\frac{1}{2}P_x+1\frac{1}{2}P_{x+1})$ when we have a census only for the middle year we are in effect off-setting a small group of deaths and net migrations represented by $(\frac{1}{2}P_x-1\frac{1}{2}P_{x+1})$ against a corresponding group represented by $(1\frac{1}{2}P_{x-1}-2\frac{1}{2}P_x)$, and the result would, no doubt, be reasonably accurate apart from age-errors. Since age-errors tend to run in quinary cycles it might well be worth while investigating the suitability of basing a table on the numbers of deaths in the 5 years surrounding the census year with the exposed-to-risk at each age computed from $(P_{x-2}+P_{x-1}+P_x+P_{x+1}+P_{x+2})$. We might then obtain pivotal values of m_x from quinary groupings of $\mathring{m}_x$ or apply some other graduation process to the individual values of $\mathring{m}_x$. It may well be that Watson adhered to King's process as closely as possible because this process was well understood and used by various workers in the field of vital statistics other than actuaries.

9·4. The oldest ages

King's process of pivotal values and osculatory interpolation does not produce rates at the youngest and oldest ages. For E.L.T. No. 10 the last pivotal values were for age 92. While the central osculatory-interpolation formula could not produce rates beyond age 87 it would have been possible to devise a suitable interpolation formula to fill in the rates for ages 88–91. This was not in fact done. After some experiments it was decided to continue the rates after age 87 by assuming that $\operatorname{colog} p_{x+5}/\operatorname{colog} p_x = r^5$, where r^5 was taken as 1·40 for males and 1·42 for females. These values of r were fixed experimentally by comparing actual and expected deaths. There is a fair agreement except that the male rates for ages 95–99 are a little on the high side.

For E.L.T. No. 8 King had completed the tables at the oldest ages by means of a fourth-difference extrapolation formula for $\log p_x$ based on the two pivotal rates at ages 91 and 96 and the interpolated rates for ages 88, 89 and 90.

For E.L.T. No. 9 Watson attempted to follow King's process at the oldest ages but found that the extrapolated rates began to decline after age 100. After some experimenting he completed the table from age 85 by a Gompertz formula obtaining the value of the common ratio from $r^{10} = \operatorname{colog} p_{94}/\operatorname{colog} p_{84}$.

9·5. The youngest ages

From the earliest days it was realized that the census figures at the youngest ages were unreliable and unsuitable for the purpose of fixing the exposed-to-risk to be applied to the deaths at these ages. It appears that for some reasons which have never been fully understood a significant number of children were omitted from the census enumerations. It is unlikely that this kind of difficulty would be significant at the present day, but the irregularities in the numbers of births from quarter to quarter would in any case render the process of mean populations based on the census enumerations unsuitable. At the infantile ages the mortality rates fall very rapidly and rates for individual ages need to be obtained directly from the data of births and deaths. For E.L.T. No. 8 King used the numbers of births recorded in the relevant years, but for E.L.T. No. 9 Watson extended the process to quarterly figures of births because of the very rapid changes in births in the relevant quarters prior to the 1921 census. A similar analysis by quarters was used for E.L.T. No. 10, and it is sufficient to give a detailed description of the process used for these latest tables. This process is a commonsense process of tracing the births as closely as possible to correspond with the deaths at the relevant age.

First, it may be noted that

$$q_0 = q_0^1 + q_0^2 + q_0^3 + q_0^4,$$

where, for example, q_0^2 is the 'probability' of dying in the second quarter of the first year of life, i.e.

$$q_0^2 = (l_{.25} - l_{.50})/l_0.$$

Watson obtained observed rates for the separate quarters of the first year of life in the following way:

$$\mathring{q}_0^1 \doteqdot \frac{\text{deaths in 1930, 1931 and 1932 under 3 months of age}}{\tfrac{1}{2}B_{29}^4 + B_{30} + B_{31} + B_{32} - \tfrac{1}{2}B_{32}^4},$$

$$\mathring{q}_0^2 \doteqdot \frac{\substack{\text{deaths in 1930, 1931 and 1932 over 3 months but} \\ \text{under 6 months of age}}}{\tfrac{1}{2}B_{29}^3 + B_{29}^4 + B_{30} + B_{31} + B_{32}^1 + B_{32}^2 + \tfrac{1}{2}B_{32}^3},$$

and so on for $\mathring{q}_0^3$ and $\mathring{q}_0^4$ where, for example, B_{30} represents the births in the year 1930 and B_{29}^3 represents the births in the third quarter of 1929.

For ages 1–5 a less meticulous process was used. The following is a typical example:

$$\mathring{q}_2 \doteqdot \frac{\text{deaths at age 2}}{\text{relevant births less relevant deaths}},$$

where (a) the 'deaths at age 2' are the deaths at that age in the years 1930, 1931 and 1932,

(b) the 'relevant births'

$$= \tfrac{1}{8}(B_{27}^1 + 3B_{27}^2 + 5B_{27}^3 + 7B_{27}^4)$$
$$+ B_{28} + B_{29}$$
$$+ \tfrac{1}{8}(7B_{30}^1 + 5B_{30}^2 + 3B_{30}^3 + B_{30}^4),$$

and (c) the 'relevant deaths' are the deaths at age 0 in 1928, 1929 and 1930 plus the deaths at age 1 in 1929, 1930 and 1931.

The application of King's method to the main part of E.L.T. No. 10 gave pivotal values at ages 12, 17, etc. Comparisons were made at each age from 6 to 16 between the census figures and the birth statistics for the relevant years and quarters. Owing to the rapid changes in the numbers of births from quarter to quarter during and immediately after the 1914–18 war, the accuracy of the pivotal values at ages 12 and 17 was open to serious doubt. Accordingly, a special process was adopted to obtain suitable rates for ages 6–16. For ages 17–22 rates were fitted in to provide a smooth junction with the rates before age 17 and after age 22.

For ages 6–16 the exposed-to-risk were obtained by a combination of the census figures and the numbers of births and deaths in the relevant preceding periods. First, an estimate was made of the number of births from which the deaths at age x last birthday in the years 1930–32 must have arisen. Taking age 12 as an example, assuming a uniform distribution of deaths over the year of age and allowing for the uneven distribution of births from quarter to quarter, Watson reached the following expression for this preliminary estimate of the relevant number of births:

$$A_{12} = \tfrac{1}{8}B_{17}^1 + \tfrac{3}{8}B_{17}^2 + \tfrac{5}{8}B_{17}^3 + \tfrac{7}{8}B_{17}^4$$
$$+ B_{18} + B_{19}$$
$$+ \tfrac{7}{8}B_{20}^1 + \tfrac{5}{8}B_{20}^2 + \tfrac{3}{8}B_{20}^3 + \tfrac{1}{8}B_{20}^4.$$

The next step was to obtain a suitable factor for adjusting A_{12} to allow for the deaths (and net migrations) between birth and exposure to death at age 12 in the 3-year period. In view of the fluctuations in the birth-rate the ratio of the census figure at age 12 to the number of births to which this figure related was not entirely suitable. Instead, Watson took the numbers enumerated at ages 11, 12 and 13 as an estimate of what the combined census figures at age 12 would have been if a census had been taken in each of the three years 1930, 1931 and 1932. The number enumerated at age 11 in 1931 was evidently a good estimate of the number aged 12 in 1932 apart from the error due to a few deaths and migrations in the intervening 12 months. Similarly, the number enumerated at age 13 in 1931 was a good estimate of the number aged 12 in 1930 apart from the corresponding error of the opposite sign.

The final step was to estimate the number of births from which the population enumerated at ages 11, 12 and 13 at the census date must have arisen. For this purpose the census date was assumed to be the end of April 1931 and Watson's estimate of the relevant number of births was as follows:

$$C_{12} = \tfrac{2}{3}B_{17}^2 + B_{17}^3 + B_{17}^4$$
$$+ B_{18} + B_{19}$$
$$+ B_{20}^1 + \tfrac{1}{3}B_{20}^2.$$

The central exposed-to-risk at age 12 was then taken as

$$E_{12}^c = \frac{A_{12}(P_{11}+P_{12}+P_{13})}{C_{12}},$$

and the rates of mortality for ages 6–16 were given by

$$\mathring{m}_x \doteqdot \frac{\text{deaths at age } x \text{ last birthday in 1930–32}}{E_x^c}.$$

These rates were subjected to a smoothing process (details un-stated) before being converted to q_x for the Life Tables.

For E.L.T. No. 8 George King had mortality rates up to age 5 based on the births and deaths figures. He also had rates from and including age 16. In addition, he had the pivotal rate at age 11. He completed the table of rates for the intervening ages by fourth-degree interpolation based on the rates at ages 4, 5, 11, 16 and 17.

For E.L.T. No. 9 the missing rates were obtained by third-difference interpolation based on the rates for ages 5, 9, 14 and 15, those for ages 9 and 14 being pivotal rates. Watson noted that these interpolated rates showed a close agreement with the (not so smooth) crude rates obtained directly from the census and deaths figures at each age.

9·6. Sectional investigations and life tables

The Registrar-General's Decennial Supplements contain much information about the mortality experience of various sections of the population and also life tables for certain geographical areas. The sectional investigations include subdivisions by geographical area, density of population, marital status, occupation, social class. The last two have been treated in considerable detail in separate volumes. Watson had long been interested in mortality analyses by geographical area, this being the basis of his sectional life tables based on the Manchester Unity Experience of 1893–97. In the 1911 Supplement life tables were given separately for each sex for the County of London, the combined County Boroughs, the combined Urban Districts and the combined Rural Districts. In the 1921 Supplement Watson made a much more extensive analysis. He subdivided the country into eleven regions and provided rates of mortality according to age-groups for each sex separately for the County Boroughs, Urban Districts and Rural Districts of each of these regions. After examination and comparison of these sectional experiences Watson constructed complete sets of rates for ages 0–84 for males and females separately for (*a*) Northumberland and Durham County Boroughs which showed the heaviest mortality, (*b*) Eastern Counties Rural Districts which showed the lightest mortality and (*c*) the County Boroughs, Urban Districts and Rural Districts respectively in the Central Counties. He also provided full life tables for Greater London. Some of these sectional tables have been fairly extensively used for actuarial purposes, particularly the Eastern Counties Rural Districts Males table for ordinary life assurance before the publication of the A 1924–29 table and for friendly societies work in combination with Manchester Unity sickness rates. The Central Counties Urban Districts Male table has also been combined with the Manchester Unity sickness rates.

In the 1931 Decennial Supplement the sectional analysis was continued on the basis of a somewhat different regional classification which had in the meantime been adopted by the Registrar-General. Group rates for quinary age-groups are given for the various geographical divisions together with comparisons with E.L.T. No. 10. Rates for individual ages 0–84 for each sex are given for the highest and lowest mortality areas, Northumberland and Durham County Boroughs and Eastern Region Rural Districts respectively. Complete life tables are again provided for Greater London.

In the 1911 Supplement separate life tables were given for single, married and widowed women. Watson discussed the suitability of combining such rates of mortality at successive ages to provide a life table and pointed out that in no circumstances could such a table have any meaning or purpose because of the decremental and incremental processes operating (and almost certainly operating selectively) to diminish and augment the numbers of lives in the respective groups. This is not the place to discuss the relative degrees of validity of the processes of construction of mortality tables based on data of different kinds and the purposes that they serve, but we can at any rate agree with Watson's view of the futility of the kind of marital-status life tables constructed in connexion with the 1911 census. This is not to say that rates of mortality at each age for single, married and widowed women separately are not a perfectly legitimate subject for investigation. In fact, such an investigation was made by Watson in the 1921 Decennial Supplement, rates for the individual ages from 16 to 84 being given for the three marital statuses separately. A similar analysis is not possible for male lives because the deaths are not subdivided for males according to marital status. Accordingly, when the mortality of married men, for example, has been required in connexion with National Insurance and for other purposes, approximations have had to be made in the light of the statistics of other countries, notably Scotland.

For the 1931 Decennial Supplement Watson provided mortality rates at quinary age-points for single, married and widowed women separately, together with various comparisons.

The subject of comparative mortality is outside the scope of this book which is concerned mainly with principles and methods. Comparative information and details about occupational mortality and other analyses are fully treated in Cox's *Demography*, where information is also given about Scottish mortality statistics.

9·7. Inter-censal population estimates and mortality rates based thereon

In recent years the Registrar-General has maintained a system of continuously adjusting the age-distributions of the population of England and Wales by reference to the births, deaths and migration statistics, and he regularly publishes estimates of the population in the various age-groups. On the basis of these estimates and the published figures for the deaths W. S. Hocking has provided in *J.I.A.* a yearly record of the mortality rates for England and Wales for the two sexes separately for quinary groups of ages. No attempt is made to adjust the group-rates to the middle ages of the groups, but the Government Actuary's Department has provided tables of mortality rates at quinary age-points for various periods in connexion with estimates for National Insurance and for the Royal

Commission on Population. Further information on these tables is given by Cox in *Demography*.

Having regard to the reliability of these inter-censal population estimates and of the mortality rates based thereon it might be thought that the construction of further English Life Tables in connexion with the census would now be unnecessary. It is true that actuaries have used the English Life Tables extensively for certain purposes, notably for the financial calculations in connexion with industrial life assurance, but this is mainly because these tables have been readily available. In their absence actuaries would no doubt readily find or construct suitable alternative tables for these purposes. It may be, however, that the series will be continued in order to provide a standard of comparison both for official and unofficial sectional investigations. For these investigations the census itself remains an indispensable instrument. While the statistics for the deaths are available year by year in age-groups for various sections of the population, the age-distribution of the corresponding sections of the population are available only from the census. Inter-censal estimates of the age-distributions of sections of the population would be of very doubtful validity because of the large element of internal migration that is going on all the time. It may be because of the need to serve the purposes of those interested in sectional experiences, such as sociologists, local government officials, medical officers of health and so on, that not only will the series of English Life Tables be continued but the methods used will continue to be on the lines introduced by George King and now so widely understood. Otherwise, it might have been useful to suggest that these national life tables serve two rather different sets of needs which ideally call for rather different treatment. The actuaries' purposes would be best served by a completely smooth table which would not need to follow the actual experience very closely in all its wave-like twists and turns. On the other hand, for the various comparative purposes a table providing a close representation of the actual experience is obviously to be desired. It might be countered that the actuaries' needs would be better served by a table based on their own insurance or other data or, perhaps better still, by hypothetical tables which recognize that the problems for which they are to be used relate to the future rather than to the present or past experience. Nevertheless, if future tables were constructed by means of a more drastic smoothing process—possibly a curve-fitting process of some kind—producing mortality rates broadly reflecting the actual experience but departing therefrom in detail over short ranges of ages, it would be desirable for close comparative purposes to provide a set of adjustments by taking out the differences between the actual and the graduated rates, and then applying some light graduation process to them such as a low-powered summation formula (i.e. a moving-average process with an adjustment for the systematic second-difference error). By adding to the main graduated rates these graduated adjustments (which would obviously oscillate around zero if the graduations were satisfactory) a closer but less smooth set of 'graduated' rates would thus be available for the purposes of close comparisons.

In this connexion it may be observed that following upon the introduction of National Health Insurance in 1911 a more up-to-date population mortality table than E.L.T. No. 6 was required to provide the basis for computing certain reserve values for the purposes of the scheme. Accordingly, estimates were made of the population living in the various age-groups corresponding to the deaths for the then most up-to-date 3-year period, 1908–10 (see *J.I.A.* **47**, 548). We need not discuss the process by which these estimates were reached. The immediate interest lies in the fact that a curve-fitting method was used to obtain the graduated table from the numbers of deaths and the estimated mean populations for denary age-groups. The numbers of deaths and the mean populations were first continuously summed, i.e. values of $\sum_t {}_0\theta_{x+t}$ and $\sum_t {}_0P_{x+t}$ were obtained for $x = 15, 25, 35, ..., 85$. For the male table it was assumed, both for the deaths and for the populations, that the logarithms of these sums could be represented by a function of the age of the form $A + Bx + Cx^2 + mr^x$. The actual fitting process is not of particular interest and need not be detailed here. It was, however, mentioned in the report on the work that before fitting the curve to the sums of the numbers of deaths they should in principle be adjusted to conform to the graduated values of ΣP_{x+t}. This was not done for the males table because the discrepancies were small. The adjustments were, however, carried out for the females table for which a further adjustment was also necessary for the graduation of the deaths at the ages below 55 where, in those days, female mortality showed certain special characteristics. The report itself is well worth reading as an example of the successful way in which a master hand such as G. F. Hardy was able to make actuarial bricks with a limited amount of suitable straw.

INDEX

Off-period, 90
Osculatory interpolation, 135–41

Pearson, K., 112
Perks, W., 10
Pivotal-value formula, 131–4
Poisson variance, 10
Policy-year experience, 15–16, 27, 28
Proportion sick, 82

Redington, F. M.: binomial test, 9,
  111; uncertainty analogy, 29
Registrar-General's estimates, 149
Retirement rates, 103–4
Revivals, 73
Risk-time, 31

Selection, 17, 78, 98, 99
Service table, 2
Sickness: definition, 81, 82; adjustments for new entrants and leavers,
  93, 94; Coward's paper, 91;
  exposed-to-risk, 92, 93; frequency
  distribution, 87; Harvey's paper, 99;
  idealization of rates, 85; Manchester

Unity Experience, 89, 90, 94, 97–9;
  off-period, 90; proportion sick, two
  forms, 82; selection, 98, 99;
  special rules, 99, 100; standard
  deviation, 88, 89; Watson's paper,
  91; waiting-period, 93
Signs, test of, 127
Sine curve for blending, 146
Sprague, T. B.: graduation of 1884
  annuitants' experience, 122, 123;
  osculatory interpolation, 138, 146
Statistics (Johnson and Tetley), 20,
  111, 115, 128, 134

Tests of graduation, 9, 125–9

Vaughan, H., 138

Waiting-period, 93
Waters, A. C., 147
Watson, Sir A. W.: English Life
  Tables Nos. 9 and 10, 150–6;
  Sickness paper, 91
Whittall, W. J. H., 40
Withdrawal rates, 101–3